Jurassic Perk

Bringing Your Inner Dinosaur Back to Life

Volodymyr Rybaiev

Table of Contents

CHAPTER 1: WELCOME TO JURASSIC PERK: YOUR DNA ISN'T FOSSILIZED YET!

Alright, folks! Grab your favorite beverage, kick back, and let's dive into the wild world of your inner dinosaur. No, we're not talking about that growling stomach of yours (though a snack might not be a bad idea). We're talking about the **real** beast within—your DNA.

You might be thinking, "DNA? Isn't that just some science-y stuff that makes me, well, me?" Yeah, sure, but it's also the blueprint that's been passed down from generation to generation, all the way back to when dinosaurs roamed the Earth. And guess what? Just like those prehistoric giants, your DNA is fighting to survive in a world that's constantly changing.

So, buckle up, because we're about to embark on a journey to unlock the secrets of cellular preservation and keep your genetic code from going the way of the dodo.

Kickstarting Your Inner Dinosaur: A User's Manual

First things first, let's get acquainted with your inner dinosaur. Now, don't go looking in the mirror expecting to see scales and sharp teeth. Your inner dinosaur is more about the **essence** of those ancient creatures—their strength, resilience, and adaptability.

Meet Your DNA

Think of your DNA as the ultimate instruction manual for your body. It's got all the info needed to make you, you—from the color of your eyes to whether you can roll your tongue (go on, try it, we'll wait). But here's the kicker: your DNA isn't just a static set of instructions. It's **alive**, constantly interacting with your environment and responding to the choices you make.

The Epigenetic Elevator Pitch

You might have heard the term "epigenetics" thrown around. It's a fancy word for how your lifestyle and environment can **turn on or off** certain genes. Imagine your DNA as a massive control panel with millions of switches. Epigenetics is like the hand that flips those switches, deciding which genes get expressed and which stay silent.

Fun Fact: Identical twins start with the exact same DNA, but as they age, their epigenetic profiles diverge. That's why one twin might develop a disease while the other stays healthy. Pretty wild, huh?

The Lowdown on Why Your Cells Are Like Prehistoric Jello

Now that we've got the basics down, let's talk about why your cells are like prehistoric jello. No, they're not wobbly and delicious (though if you've ever seen a cell under a microscope, they do look pretty jiggly). What we mean is that your cells, much like those ancient single-celled organisms, are constantly adapting to their environment.

The Cellular Time Capsule

Your cells are like tiny time capsules, carrying genetic information that's been passed down for millions of years. But here's the thing: while your DNA might be ancient, your cells are constantly renewing themselves. In fact, **most of your cells are younger than you are**. Mind-blowing, right?

The Aging Process: A Dino's Tale

So, if your cells are constantly renewing, why do you age? Well, think of it like a game of telephone. Each time your cells divide, they pass along a copy of your DNA. But with each copy, there's a chance for mistakes—mutations that can accumulate over time.

Plus, as you age, your cells become less efficient at repairing damage and clearing out waste. It's like your cellular janitorial staff starts taking longer coffee breaks. The result? A buildup of cellular gunk that can lead to everything from wrinkles to chronic diseases.

The Jurassic Perk Philosophy

But here's where the **Jurassic Perk philosophy** comes in. Just because aging is inevitable doesn't mean you can't slow it down and age **well**. By understanding the science behind cellular preservation and making smart lifestyle choices, you can keep your DNA from going extinct before its time.

The Power of Prevention

You know the saying, "An ounce of prevention is worth a pound of cure"? Well, that's especially true when it comes to your DNA. By taking care of your cells **now**, you can prevent a whole host of issues down the line.

The Dino Mindset

But Jurassic Perk isn't just about what you do—it's about how you **think**. It's about embracing the dino mindset: strong, resilient, and adaptable. It's about seeing every challenge as an opportunity to grow and every setback as a chance to learn.

Your Jurassic Journey Awaits

So, are you ready to embark on this prehistoric adventure? To dive deep into the world of cellular preservation and unlock the secrets of your inner dinosaur? Then grab your metaphorical pith helmet and let's get started.

In the coming chapters, we'll explore everything from the **science of aging** to the **power of nutrition**. We'll talk about **exercise, stress management**, and even **dino-proofing your environment**. And we'll do it all with a healthy dose of humor, because let's face it, life's too short to take everything seriously.

A Word of Warning

Now, before we dive in, a word of warning: this isn't your typical self-help book. We're not promising a quick fix or a magic pill. What we **are** promising is a journey—a journey of self-discovery, growth, and empowerment. And like any good journey, it's going to take time, effort, and maybe even a few wrong turns.

But don't worry, we'll be here every step of the way, cheering you on and offering a helping hand when you need it. Because at the end of the day, we're all in this together. We're all just dinosaurs trying to make it in a modern world.

CHAPTER 2: THE DINO-MITE GUIDE TO CELLULAR PRESERVATION

Alright, folks! You've got your inner dinosaur all revved up and ready to go. Now it's time to dive into the nitty-gritty of cellular preservation. Think of this chapter as your ultimate guide to keeping your cells happy, healthy, and ready to roar.

Unraveling the Mysteries of Your Cellular Time Capsule

Before we get into the how-to's, let's take a closer look at what's going on inside those tiny time capsules we call cells. After all, understanding the problem is the first step to solving it.

The Cellular Blueprint

Remember how we talked about DNA being the blueprint for your body? Well, each of your cells contains a copy of that blueprint, tucked away in a little structure called the **nucleus**. But here's the thing: not every cell uses the entire blueprint.

Think of it like building a house. You've got the blueprint for the whole thing, but you don't need to know about the plumbing when you're working on the electrical system. In the same way, your cells only **express** the genes they need to do their specific jobs.

The Epigenetic Orchestra

Now, you might be wondering, "How do cells know which genes to express?" That's where **epigenetics** comes in. Remember our control panel with millions of switches? Well, those switches are controlled by a complex system of chemical tags that attach to your DNA and the proteins it's wrapped around.

These tags act like conductors, directing the symphony of gene expression. They tell your cells which genes to turn on and which to turn off, based on signals from your environment and lifestyle. Pretty cool, huh?

How to Keep Your Cells from Turning into Dino Dust

Now that we've got a better understanding of what's going on inside our cells, let's talk about how to keep them from turning into dino dust. Hint: it's not just about slathering on the sunscreen (though that's important too).

The Four Horsemen of Cellular Aging

When it comes to cellular aging, there are four main culprits we need to watch out for. Think of them as the **Four Horsemen of Cellular Aging**:

1. **Oxidative Stress**: This is what happens when there's an imbalance between free radicals (reactive molecules that can damage cells) and antioxidants (molecules that neutralize free radicals) in your body. Think of it like a game of tug-of-war. Too much oxidative stress can lead to cell damage and accelerated aging.

2. **Inflammation**: Inflammation is your body's response to injury or infection. It's a good thing when it's acute (short-term), but chronic (long-term) inflammation can wreak havoc on your cells, leading to everything from wrinkles to heart disease.

3. **Glycation**: This is what happens when sugar molecules bind to proteins, lipids, or nucleic acids without the help of an enzyme. The result is a hodgepodge of molecules called advanced glycation end products (AGEs), which can crosslink with other proteins and cause cellular damage.

4. **DNA Damage**: Remember how we talked about mutations accumulating over time? Well, DNA damage is what happens when those mutations start to interfere with your cells' ability to function properly. It can be caused by everything from UV radiation to environmental toxins.

The Dino Defense Strategy

So, how do we fight back against these Four Horsemen? By building up our **Dino Defense Strategy**. This is a multi-pronged approach that involves everything from what we eat to how we manage stress. Let's break it down.

The Jurassic Diet: Feeding Your Inner Dinosaur

You are what you eat, right? Well, so are your cells. The food you put into your body has a direct impact on your cellular health. So, let's talk about how to feed your inner dinosaur.

The Power of Plants

When it comes to cellular preservation, plants are your best friends. They're packed with **antioxidants**, which help combat oxidative stress, and **phytonutrients**, which help fight inflammation and boost your immune system.

Pro Tip: Aim for a **rainbow** of colors on your plate. Different colored fruits and veggies contain different phytonutrients, so the more colors you eat, the more benefits you get.

The Lowdown on Macros

Macronutrients, or **macros** for short, are the big three nutrients that provide your body with energy: carbohydrates, proteins, and fats. Each one plays a crucial role in cellular health.

- **Carbohydrates**: These are your body's primary source of energy. But not all carbs are created equal. Complex carbs, like those found in whole grains and starchy vegetables, provide sustained energy and are packed with nutrients. Simple carbs, like those found in processed foods and sugary drinks, can lead to spikes in blood sugar and contribute to glycation.

- **Proteins**: Proteins are the building blocks of your cells. They're essential for everything from muscle repair to immune function. Aim for a variety of protein sources, including both animal and plant-based options.

- **Fats**: Fats are crucial for cellular health. They help maintain the integrity of your cell membranes, absorb fat-soluble vitamins, and regulate hormones. But again, not all fats are created equal. Focus on healthy fats, like those found in avocados, nuts, seeds, and fatty fish.

The Sugar Showdown

We've all heard that sugar is bad for us, but do you know why? It's not just about the calories. Sugar is a major contributor to **glycation**, which, as we talked about earlier, can lead to cellular damage and accelerated aging.

But here's the thing: not all sugars are created equal. Natural sugars, like those found in fruits, come packaged with fiber, vitamins, and minerals that slow down their absorption and mitigate their effects on your body. Added sugars, on the other hand, are often found in processed foods and can lead to rapid spikes in blood sugar.

Pro Tip: Read your labels. Added sugars can hide under a variety of names, from high fructose corn syrup to dextrose to maltose. If it ends in "-ose," it's probably a sugar.

The Hydration Station

Water is essential for cellular health. It helps transport nutrients, remove waste, and maintain the balance of electrolytes in your body. Plus, it's a key component of your cells' cytoplasm, the jelly-like substance that fills your cells.

Pro Tip: Aim for **eight 8-ounce glasses of water a day**. But remember, that's just a guideline. Your hydration needs can vary based on your activity level, climate, and overall health.

The Fitness Factor: Exercising Your Inner Dinosaur

We all know that exercise is good for us. It helps us maintain a healthy weight, boosts our mood, and keeps our hearts happy. But did you know that it also plays a crucial role in cellular preservation?

The Mitochondrial Makeover

Remember those little powerhouses we talked about earlier? The ones that produce energy for your cells? Well, exercise can actually **increase the number and efficiency of your mitochondria**. This not only boosts your energy levels but also helps combat oxidative stress and inflammation.

The Telomere Tango

Telomeres are the protective caps at the ends of your chromosomes. Think of them like the plastic tips at the ends of your shoelaces. Each time your cells divide, your telomeres get a little bit shorter. Once they reach a certain length, your cells can no longer divide, and they eventually die.

But here's the cool part: **exercise can actually slow down telomere shortening**. Studies have shown that people who exercise regularly have longer telomeres than those who don't. So, if you want to keep your cells young and healthy, it's time to get moving.

The Dino Workout Plan

So, what kind of exercise should you be doing? The answer is: **a mix of everything**.

- **Cardio**: Cardiovascular exercise, like running, cycling, or swimming, gets your heart pumping and boosts your circulation. This helps deliver oxygen and nutrients to your cells and remove waste products.

- **Strength Training**: Strength training, like weightlifting or bodyweight exercises, helps build and maintain muscle mass. This not only makes you stronger but also boosts your metabolism and helps combat age-related muscle loss.

- **Flexibility and Mobility**: Flexibility and mobility exercises, like yoga or stretching, help keep your joints and muscles limber. This not only improves your range of motion but also helps prevent injuries.

- **Balance and Coordination**: Balance and coordination exercises, like tai chi or dance, help improve your proprioception—your body's ability to sense its position in space. This not only improves your athletic performance but also helps prevent falls and injuries.

Pro Tip: Find activities you **enjoy**. The best exercise is the one you'll actually do. So, whether it's dancing, hiking, or playing pickleball, find something that brings you joy and makes you want to move.

The Sleep Solution: Resting Your Inner Dinosaur

Sleep is often overlooked when it comes to health and wellness. But the truth is, **sleep is essential for cellular preservation**. Here's why.

The Cellular Clean-Up Crew

Remember how we talked about your cellular janitorial staff taking longer coffee breaks as you age? Well, sleep is when they do their best work. During sleep, your body goes into repair mode, clearing out waste products, repairing damaged cells, and producing growth hormones.

The Hormonal Harmony

Sleep also plays a crucial role in regulating your hormones. It helps balance your hunger and satiety hormones, ghrelin and leptin, which can help prevent overeating and weight gain. It also helps regulate your stress hormones, like cortisol, which can help combat inflammation and oxidative stress.

The Memory Matrix

But sleep isn't just about physical health. It's also crucial for cognitive function. During sleep, your brain consolidates memories, clears out waste products, and forms new neural connections. This not only improves your memory and learning but also helps prevent cognitive decline as you age.

The Dino Dream Plan

So, how can you optimize your sleep for cellular preservation? Here are some tips:

- **Consistency is Key**: Try to go to bed and wake up at the same time every day, even on weekends. This helps regulate your body's internal clock and makes it easier to fall asleep and stay asleep.

- **Create a Sleep Sanctuary**: Make your bedroom a haven for sleep. Keep it cool, dark, and quiet, and invest in a comfortable mattress and pillows.

- **Power Down**: Avoid screens before bed. The blue light emitted by phones, tablets, and TVs can interfere with your body's production of melatonin, a hormone that regulates sleep.

- **Wind Down**: Establish a relaxing bedtime routine. This could include reading, taking a warm bath, or practicing relaxation exercises like deep breathing or meditation.

- **Watch What You Eat and Drink**: Avoid large meals, caffeine, and alcohol close to bedtime. All of these can interfere with your sleep quality.

Pro Tip: Aim for **7-9 hours of sleep per night**. But remember, quality is just as important as quantity. If you're not waking up feeling rested, it might be time to reassess your sleep habits.

The Stress Solution: Soothing Your Inner Dinosaur

Stress is a fact of life. Whether it's work deadlines, family drama, or just the daily grind, we all face stress on a regular basis. But while a little bit of stress can be a good thing (it can boost your immune system and enhance your performance), too much stress can wreak havoc on your cells.

The Fight or Flight Response

When you're stressed, your body goes into **fight or flight mode**. This is an evolutionary response designed to help you deal with immediate threats, like, say, a hungry T-Rex. Your heart rate increases, your blood pressure goes up, and your body pumps out stress hormones like cortisol and adrenaline.

But here's the thing: while this response is great for dealing with short-term threats, it's not so great when it's constantly activated. Chronic stress can lead to everything from high blood pressure to weakened immunity to accelerated aging.

The Inflammation Connection

One of the ways stress affects your cells is through **inflammation**. When you're stressed, your body produces inflammatory cytokines, which are like little chemical messengers that tell your immune system to ramp up its response.

But while a little bit of inflammation can be a good thing (it helps your body fight off infections and heal from injuries), too much inflammation can lead to cellular damage and accelerated aging.

The Dino De-Stress Plan

So, how can you combat stress and keep your inner dinosaur happy and healthy? Here are some tips:

- **Mindfulness and Meditation**: Practices like mindfulness and meditation can help you stay present and reduce stress. They can also help lower your blood pressure, improve your immune function, and even slow down telomere shortening.

- **Exercise**: We've already talked about the benefits of exercise for cellular health. But did you know that it's also a great stress buster? Exercise helps reduce stress hormones and increases the production of endorphins, your body's natural mood boosters.

- **Social Support**: Connecting with others can be a powerful stress reliever. Whether it's spending time with friends and family, joining a club or group, or volunteering in your community, social support can help buffer the effects of stress.

- **Self-Care**: Taking care of yourself is crucial for managing stress. This could include anything from getting a massage to taking a warm bath to indulging in your favorite hobby. Whatever brings you joy and helps you relax, make time for it.

- **Boundaries**: Learn to say no. It's okay to have limits and to prioritize your own needs. Whether it's setting boundaries at work or learning to delegate tasks, don't be afraid to advocate for yourself.

Pro Tip: Stress management is a **personal** thing. What works for one person might not work for another. The key is to find what works for you and make it a regular part of your routine.

The Environmental Element: Dino-Proofing Your Habitat

Your environment plays a crucial role in your cellular health. From the air you breathe to the products you use, everything in your environment has the potential to affect your cells. So, let's talk about how to **dino-proof your habitat.**

The Air You Breathe

The air you breathe can have a big impact on your cellular health. Pollutants, allergens, and other irritants can cause oxidative stress, inflammation, and even DNA damage.

Pro Tip: Invest in an **air purifier** for your home. Look for one with a HEPA filter, which can remove up to 99.97% of airborne particles. Also, consider adding some **houseplants** to your space. Plants like snake plants, spider plants, and peace lilies are known for their air-purifying properties.

The Water You Drink

The water you drink is another important factor in your cellular health. While tap water is generally safe to drink, it can contain contaminants like chlorine, lead, and even pharmaceutical residues.

Pro Tip: Consider investing in a **water filter** for your home. Look for one that's certified by the National Sanitation Foundation (NSF) to remove a wide range of contaminants.

The Products You Use

The products you use on your body and in your home can also affect your cellular health. Many personal care and cleaning products contain chemicals that can disrupt your hormones, cause oxidative stress, and even damage your DNA.

Pro Tip: Opt for **natural and organic products** whenever possible. Look for products that are free from parabens, phthalates, sulfates, and other harmful chemicals. Also, consider making your own cleaning products using natural ingredients like vinegar, baking soda, and essential oils.

The Radiation Rundown

Radiation is a fact of life. It comes from the sun, the earth, and even the food we eat. But while a little bit of radiation is unavoidable, too much can be harmful.

Pro Tip: Limit your exposure to **electromagnetic radiation** from devices like cell phones, computers, and Wi-Fi routers.

Turn off your devices when you're not using them, and consider using a landline for long phone calls. Also, be sure to wear sunscreen and protective clothing when you're out in the sun to protect yourself from **UV radiation**.

The Dino Detox Plan

So, how can you detox your environment and keep your inner dinosaur happy and healthy? Here are some tips:

- **Green Your Space**: Fill your home with plants. Not only do they purify the air, but they also add a touch of nature to your space.

- **Ditch the Plastic**: Opt for glass, stainless steel, or ceramic containers instead of plastic. Plastic can leach harmful chemicals into your food and drinks, especially when heated.

- **Go Organic**: Choose organic foods whenever possible. Organic foods are grown without the use of synthetic pesticides, fertilizers, or GMOs, which can be harmful to your cells.

- **Filter Your Water**: Invest in a water filter for your home. Look for one that's certified to remove a wide range of contaminants.

- **Clean Green**: Use natural and organic cleaning products. Look for products that are free from harmful chemicals, or consider making your own using natural ingredients.

Pro Tip: Detoxing your environment is a **process**. Don't try to do it all at once. Start with one or two changes and build from there.

CHAPTER 3: DNA DON'TS: EXTINCTION-LEVEL EVENTS YOU CAN AVOID

Alright, folks! We've talked about the importance of cellular preservation and how to keep your inner dinosaur roaring. Now it's time to dive into the **DNA Don'ts**—those extinction-level events you can avoid to keep your genetic code from going the way of the dodo.

The Top 10 Ways You're Aging Your DNA Like a T-Rex in a Tar Pit

Let's face it, life is full of pitfalls that can accelerate aging and damage your DNA. But the good news is, many of these pitfalls are avoidable. So, let's talk about the top 10 ways you might be aging your DNA like a T-Rex in a tar pit— and how to steer clear of them.

1. Smoking: The DNA Disaster

We all know that smoking is bad for us. But do you know why? Smoking introduces a **cocktail of chemicals** into your body that can cause oxidative stress, inflammation, and even DNA damage. Plus, it accelerates telomere shortening, which, as we talked about earlier, is a major contributor to cellular aging.

Pro Tip: If you smoke, **quitting is the single best thing you can do for your health.** Talk to your doctor about quitting strategies that might work for you.

2. Sugar Overload: The Glycation Game

We've already talked about the dangers of sugar and glycation. But it's worth repeating: too much sugar can wreak havoc on your cells, leading to everything from wrinkles to chronic diseases.

Pro Tip: Limit your intake of added sugars. Opt for natural sugars found in fruits and veggies, and be sure to read your labels. Remember, if it ends in "-ose," it's probably a sugar.

3. Sun Worshipping: The UV Dilemma

The sun is a double-edged sword. On one hand, it provides essential vitamin D. On the other hand, it emits **UV radiation**, which can cause DNA damage, oxidative stress, and even skin cancer.

Pro Tip: Wear sunscreen every day, even on cloudy days. Opt for a broad-spectrum sunscreen with an SPF of at least 30. Also, consider wearing protective clothing and seeking shade during peak sun hours.

4. Sedentary Lifestyle: The Couch Potato Conundrum

A sedentary lifestyle is a major contributor to accelerated aging. Not only does it lead to weight gain and muscle loss, but it also increases your risk of chronic diseases like heart disease, diabetes, and even some cancers.

Pro Tip: Get moving. Aim for at least **30 minutes of moderate-intensity exercise most days of the week**. But remember, every little bit counts. Even a short walk around the block can make a difference.

5. Stress Overload: The Cortisol Crisis

We've talked about the dangers of chronic stress and how it can lead to inflammation, oxidative stress, and even DNA damage. But it's worth repeating: too much stress is a **major** contributor to accelerated aging.

Pro Tip: Find ways to manage stress. Whether it's meditation, exercise, or spending time with loved ones, find what works for you and make it a regular part of your routine.

6. Sleep Deprivation: The Insomnia Issue

Sleep is essential for cellular repair and regeneration. But too many of us are burning the candle at both ends, leading to sleep deprivation and all the health issues that come with it.

Pro Tip: Prioritize sleep. Aim for **7-9 hours of quality sleep per night**. Establish a relaxing bedtime routine, create a sleep sanctuary, and avoid screens before bed.

7. Substance Abuse: The Chemical Cocktail

Substance abuse, whether it's alcohol, drugs, or even prescription medications, can wreak havoc on your cells. It can lead to oxidative stress, inflammation, and even DNA damage.

Pro Tip: Limit your intake of alcohol and avoid illicit drugs. If you're struggling with substance abuse, talk to your doctor about treatment options.

8. Poor Diet: The Nutrient Nightmare

A poor diet can accelerate aging and lead to a host of health issues. But the good news is, it's never too late to turn things around.

Pro Tip: Eat a balanced diet rich in fruits, veggies, whole grains, lean proteins, and healthy fats. Limit your intake of processed foods, sugary drinks, and unhealthy fats.

9. Environmental Toxins: The Chemical Conundrum

From the air we breathe to the products we use, our environment is full of toxins that can damage our cells. But the good news is, there are steps we can take to limit our exposure.

Pro Tip: Detox your environment. Opt for natural and organic products, filter your water, and invest in an air purifier for your home.

10. Negative Thinking: The Mindset Muddle

Believe it or not, your thoughts can have a **profound impact** on your cellular health. Negative thinking can lead to stress, inflammation, and even DNA damage.

Pro Tip: Cultivate a positive mindset. Practice gratitude, focus on the good in your life, and surround yourself with positive people.

Steering Clear of Genetic Potholes: A Survival Guide

Now that we've talked about the top 10 ways you might be aging your DNA, let's dive deeper into some **genetic potholes** you can avoid—and how to steer clear of them.

The Alcohol Adventure

Alcohol is a tricky one. On one hand, moderate alcohol consumption has been linked to a **reduced risk of heart disease**. On the other hand, excessive alcohol consumption can lead to a host of health issues, including liver disease, brain damage, and even some cancers.

Pro Tip: Everything in moderation. If you choose to drink, **limit your intake to one drink per day for women and two drinks per day for men**. And remember, a standard drink is smaller than you might think: 12 ounces of beer, 5 ounces of wine, or 1.5 ounces of distilled spirits.

The Drug Dilemma

Illicit drugs are a **major** contributor to accelerated aging. They can cause oxidative stress, inflammation, and even DNA damage. Plus, they can lead to addiction, which can wreak havoc on your life and your health.

Pro Tip: Just say no. If you're struggling with drug addiction, talk to your doctor about treatment options.

The Prescription Puzzle

Prescription medications can be a **lifesaver** for many people. But they can also come with a host of side effects, including accelerated aging.

Pro Tip: Talk to your doctor. If you're concerned about the side effects of your medications, talk to your doctor about alternatives. And always **follow the dosage instructions** on your prescription.

The Air Quality Quandary

Air pollution is a **major** contributor to accelerated aging. It can cause oxidative stress, inflammation, and even DNA damage.

Pro Tip: Invest in an air purifier for your home. Look for one with a HEPA filter, which can remove up to 99.97% of airborne particles. Also, consider adding some **houseplants** to your space. Plants like snake plants, spider plants, and peace lilies are known for their air-purifying properties.

The Water Worry

Water pollution is another **major** contributor to accelerated aging. It can introduce a host of toxins into your body, including heavy metals, pesticides, and even pharmaceutical residues.

Pro Tip: Filter your water. Look for a water filter that's certified by the National Sanitation Foundation (NSF) to remove a wide range of contaminants.

The Chemical Concern

Chemicals are **everywhere**—in our food, our personal care products, our cleaning supplies, even our furniture. And many of these chemicals can damage our cells and accelerate aging.

Pro Tip: Opt for natural and organic products whenever possible. Look for products that are free from parabens, phthalates, sulfates, and other harmful chemicals. Also, consider making your own cleaning products using natural ingredients like vinegar, baking soda, and essential oils.

The Radiation Rundown

Radiation is a fact of life. It comes from the sun, the earth, and even the food we eat. But while a little bit of radiation is unavoidable, too much can be harmful.

Pro Tip: Limit your exposure to electromagnetic radiation from devices like cell phones, computers, and Wi-Fi routers. Turn off your devices when you're not using them, and consider using a landline for long phone calls. Also, be sure to wear sunscreen and protective clothing when you're out in the sun to protect yourself from **UV radiation**.

The Mindset Muddle

Your mindset can have a **profound impact** on your cellular health. Negative thinking can lead to stress, inflammation, and even DNA damage.

Pro Tip: Cultivate a positive mindset. Practice gratitude, focus on the good in your life, and surround yourself with positive people. Also, consider practices like mindfulness and meditation, which can help you stay present and reduce stress.

CHAPTER 4: THE JURASSIC DIET: FEEDING YOUR INNER DINOSAUR

Alright, folks! We've talked about the importance of cellular preservation, the DNA don'ts, and now it's time to dive into the **Jurassic Diet**. Think of this chapter as your ultimate guide to feeding your inner dinosaur and keeping your cells happy, healthy, and ready to roar.

Chowing Down Like a Herbivore: The Plant-Powered Path

Let's face it, plants are the **real MVPs** when it comes to nutrition. They're packed with vitamins, minerals, antioxidants, and phytonutrients—all the good stuff your cells need to thrive. So, let's talk about how to **chow down like a herbivore** and reap the benefits of a plant-powered diet.

The Power of Plants

Plants are **nutritional powerhouses**. They're loaded with essential vitamins and minerals that your body needs to function properly. But that's not all. Plants also contain **phytonutrients**—powerful compounds that can help combat oxidative stress, reduce inflammation, and even protect your DNA.

Fun Fact: There are over **25,000** different phytonutrients found in plants. Talk about a nutritional treasure trove!

The Fiber Factor

Fiber is a **big deal** when it comes to cellular health. It helps keep your digestive system running smoothly, promotes healthy gut bacteria, and can even help lower cholesterol and stabilize blood sugar. Plus, it keeps you feeling full and satisfied, which can help with weight management.

Pro Tip: Aim for **25-35 grams of fiber per day**. Foods high in fiber include fruits, vegetables, whole grains, nuts, seeds, and legumes.

The Rainbow Connection

When it comes to fruits and veggies, **color matters**. Different colored produce contains different phytonutrients, each with its own unique health benefits. So, the more colors you eat, the more benefits you get.

Pro Tip: Aim for a **rainbow of colors** on your plate. Think red bell peppers, orange carrots, yellow squash, green spinach, blueberries, and purple cabbage. The more colorful your plate, the better!

The Leafy Greens Lowdown

Leafy greens are the **superstars** of the plant world. They're packed with vitamins, minerals, and antioxidants, and they're low in calories and high in fiber. Plus, they're incredibly versatile—you can eat them raw, cooked, or blended into a smoothie.

Pro Tip: Aim for **at least one serving of leafy greens per day**. Some of the best options include spinach, kale, collard greens, Swiss chard, and arugula.

Carnivore Cravings: How to Eat Meat Without Going Extinct

Now, we're not saying you have to go full-on herbivore to be healthy. Meat can be a **great source** of protein, vitamins, and minerals. But it's all about **balance** and

quality. So, let's talk about how to **satisfy your carnivore cravings** without going extinct.

The Protein Puzzle

Protein is **essential** for cellular health. It's the building block of your cells, and it plays a crucial role in everything from muscle repair to immune function. But not all protein is created equal.

Pro Tip: Opt for **lean sources of protein**, like chicken, turkey, fish, eggs, and plant-based options like beans, lentils, and tofu. Limit your intake of red meat and processed meats, which can be high in saturated fats and harmful compounds.

The Quality Conundrum

When it comes to meat, **quality matters**. The way an animal is raised can have a **big impact** on its nutritional profile. Animals raised on pasture tend to have higher levels of omega-3 fatty acids, vitamin E, and other beneficial nutrients.

Pro Tip: Choose **grass-fed, pasture-raised, and organic meat** whenever possible. Look for labels that indicate the animal was raised humanely and without the use of antibiotics or hormones.

The Portion Predicament

Portion size is a **big deal** when it comes to meat. While meat can be a great source of nutrition, too much of a good thing can be, well, not so good. Large portions of meat can lead to excess calories, saturated fat, and even increased risk of chronic diseases.

Pro Tip: Aim for **3-4 ounces of meat per serving**, about the size of a deck of cards. And remember, you don't have to have meat at every meal. Mix it up with plant-based protein sources to keep things interesting and balanced.

The Fishy Business

Fish is a **fantastic source** of protein, omega-3 fatty acids, and other beneficial nutrients. But not all fish are created equal. Some fish are high in mercury and other contaminants, which can be harmful to your health.

Pro Tip: Opt for **low-mercury fish**, like salmon, cod, haddock, and tilapia. Limit your intake of high-mercury fish, like swordfish, shark, and king mackerel. And always **cook your fish thoroughly** to kill any bacteria or parasites.

The Fat Facts: The Good, the Bad, and the Ugly

Fat is a **hot topic** when it comes to nutrition. Some people swear by low-fat diets, while others sing the praises of high-fat, low-carb plans. But the truth is, fat is **essential** for cellular health—as long as you're eating the right kinds.

The Good Fats

Good fats are the ones that **benefit your health**. They help maintain the integrity of your cell membranes, absorb fat-soluble vitamins, and regulate hormones. Plus, they can help reduce inflammation, lower cholesterol, and even improve brain function.

Pro Tip: Incorporate **healthy fats** into your diet. Some of the best sources include avocados, nuts, seeds, olive oil, and fatty fish like salmon and mackerel.

The Bad Fats

Bad fats are the ones that **harm your health**. They can increase inflammation, raise cholesterol, and even contribute to chronic diseases like heart disease and diabetes.

Pro Tip: Limit your intake of **saturated fats**, found in red meat, full-fat dairy, and tropical oils like coconut and palm oil. And avoid **trans fats** altogether, found in processed foods, fried foods, and some margarines.

The Ugly Truth About Sugar

We've talked about the dangers of sugar before, but it's worth repeating: too much sugar can wreak havoc on your cells. It can cause oxidative stress, inflammation, and even DNA damage. Plus, it can lead to weight gain, insulin resistance, and a host of other health issues.

Pro Tip: Limit your intake of added sugars. Opt for natural sugars found in fruits and veggies, and be sure to read your labels. Remember, if it ends in "-ose," it's probably a sugar.

The Carb Conundrum: The Lowdown on Carbohydrates

Carbohydrates are a **major player** in the nutrition game. They're your body's primary source of energy, and they play a crucial role in everything from brain function to athletic performance. But not all carbs are created equal.

The Good Carbs

Good carbs are the ones that **benefit your health**. They provide sustained energy, promote healthy digestion, and are packed with vitamins, minerals, and fiber.

Pro Tip: Opt for **complex carbohydrates**, like whole grains, starchy vegetables, and legumes. These carbs are digested slowly, providing steady energy and helping to stabilize blood sugar.

The Bad Carbs

Bad carbs are the ones that **harm your health**. They provide quick energy but can lead to spikes in blood sugar, insulin resistance, and even weight gain.

Pro Tip: Limit your intake of **simple carbohydrates**, like white bread, pasta, rice, and sugary drinks. These carbs are digested quickly, leading to rapid spikes in blood sugar and insulin.

The Hydration Station: The Importance of Water

Water is **essential** for cellular health. It helps transport nutrients, remove waste, and maintain the balance of electrolytes in your body. Plus, it's a key component of your cells' cytoplasm, the jelly-like substance that fills your cells.

The Dehydration Dilemma

Dehydration is a **big deal**. It can lead to fatigue, headaches, constipation, and even impaired cognitive function. Plus, it can exacerbate the effects of aging, making you look and feel older than you are.

Pro Tip: Stay hydrated. Aim for **eight 8-ounce glasses of water a day**. But remember, that's just a guideline. Your hydration needs can vary based on your activity level, climate, and overall health.

The Electrolyte Equation

Electrolytes are **minerals** that play a crucial role in your body's functioning. They help regulate fluid balance, nerve and muscle function, and even blood pressure. But when you sweat, you lose electrolytes, which can lead to dehydration and other health issues.

Pro Tip: Replace lost electrolytes with foods rich in sodium, potassium, magnesium, and calcium. Some good options include bananas, avocados, leafy greens, and nuts. And if you're sweating a lot, consider an electrolyte drink to help replenish what you've lost.

The Gut-Brain Connection: The Microbiome Matters

Your gut is home to **trillions** of bacteria, collectively known as the **microbiome**. These tiny critters play a **huge role** in your overall health, affecting everything from digestion to immune function to even your mood.

The Good Bugs

Good bacteria are the ones that **benefit your health.** They help digest food, produce vitamins, and even fight off harmful pathogens. Plus, they can help reduce inflammation, boost your immune system, and even improve your mood.

Pro Tip: Feed your good bacteria with **prebiotic foods**, like fruits, vegetables, whole grains, and legumes. These foods contain fiber that your good bacteria love to munch on.

The Bad Bugs

Bad bacteria are the ones that **harm your health.** They can cause digestive issues, inflammation, and even contribute to chronic diseases like obesity and diabetes.

Pro Tip: Starve your bad bacteria by **limiting your intake of processed foods, sugary drinks, and unhealthy fats**. These foods feed the bad bacteria, allowing them to proliferate and wreak havoc on your gut.

The Probiotic Puzzle

Probiotics are **live bacteria** that can **benefit your health.** They can help restore the balance of good bacteria in your gut, improve digestion, boost your immune system, and even reduce inflammation.

Pro Tip: Incorporate probiotic foods into your diet. Some good options include yogurt, kefir, sauerkraut, kimchi, and kombucha. And if you're not a fan of fermented foods, consider a probiotic supplement to help boost your gut health.

The Meal Planning Masterclass: Putting It All Together

Now that we've talked about the importance of plants, the quality of meat, the fat facts, the carb conundrum, the hydration station, and the gut-brain connection, it's time to put it all together into a **meal planning masterclass**.

The Breakfast Bonanza

Breakfast is the **most important meal of the day**. It sets the tone for your entire day, providing the energy and nutrients you need to tackle whatever comes your way.

Pro Tip: Start your day with a nutritious breakfast. Some good options include oatmeal with berries and nuts, a veggie-packed omelet, or a smoothie bowl with your favorite fruits and toppings.

The Lunchtime Lineup

Lunch is a **great opportunity** to pack in the nutrients and fuel your body for the afternoon ahead. But it's also a time when many of us fall into the trap of convenience foods, which can be high in calories and low in nutrition.

Pro Tip: Plan ahead and **pack a nutritious lunch**. Some good options include a salad with grilled chicken and veggies, a turkey and avocado wrap, or a quinoa bowl with roasted vegetables and chickpeas.

The Dinner Dilemma

Dinner is a **chance to unwind** and enjoy a delicious meal with friends and family. But it's also a time when many of us overindulge, leading to excess calories and digestive discomfort.

Pro Tip: Keep it light and **focus on quality**. Some good options include grilled fish with steamed vegetables, a stir-fry with tofu and colorful veggies, or a baked sweet potato with black beans and avocado.

The Snack Attack

Snacks are a **great way** to keep your energy up and your hunger at bay between meals. But it's important to choose snacks that are **nutritious** and **satisfying**.

Pro Tip: Opt for snacks that are **high in protein and fiber**. Some good options include apple slices with almond butter, carrot sticks with hummus, or a handful of nuts and dried fruit.

The Meal Prep Magic

Meal prepping is a **game-changer** when it comes to healthy eating. It saves time, reduces stress, and ensures that you always have nutritious meals on hand.

Pro Tip: Set aside time each week to **plan and prep your meals**. Choose a day that works for you, whether it's Sunday afternoon or Wednesday evening, and use that time to chop veggies, cook proteins, and portion out your meals for the week.

CHAPTER 5: FITNESS FOR DINOSAURS: EXERCISES TO KEEP YOU FROM GOING THE WAY OF THE DODO

Alright, folks! You've got your diet dialed in, and now it's time to talk about **fitness**. Think of this chapter as your ultimate guide to keeping your inner dinosaur strong, agile, and ready to roar. Whether you're a seasoned athlete or a total newbie, we've got you covered.

Moving Like a Velociraptor: Agility and Strength Training

Let's face it, velociraptors were the **ultimate athletes** of the dinosaur world. They were fast, agile, and strong—all qualities we could use a little more of in our own lives. So, let's talk about how to **move like a velociraptor** and reap the benefits of agility and strength training.

The Agility Advantage

Agility is all about **quickness** and **grace**. It's the ability to change direction, start and stop suddenly, and maintain balance and control. And it's not just for athletes—agility is crucial for everyday life, from navigating crowded sidewalks to chasing after your kids (or pets).

Pro Tip: Incorporate agility drills into your workout routine. Some good options include ladder drills, cone drills, and jump rope. These exercises not only improve your agility but also get your heart pumping and burn calories.

The Strength Solution

Strength training is a **must** for anyone looking to improve their overall fitness. It helps build and maintain muscle mass, boosts your metabolism, and even improves bone density. Plus, it makes everyday tasks, like carrying groceries or climbing stairs, a whole lot easier.

Pro Tip: Focus on compound movements that work multiple muscle groups at once. Some good options include squats, deadlifts, lunges, push-ups, and pull-ups. And remember, you don't need a fancy gym membership to get strong— bodyweight exercises and simple equipment like dumbbells and resistance bands can be just as effective.

The Full-Body Workout

Full-body workouts are a **great way** to build strength and improve overall fitness. They work multiple muscle groups at once, saving you time and maximizing your results. Plus, they can be done anywhere, with minimal equipment.

Pro Tip: Create a full-body workout that includes exercises for your upper body, lower body, and core. Aim for **3-4 sets of 8-12 reps** for each exercise, with a minute or two of rest in between. And don't forget to warm up before you start and cool down afterwards.

The Lazy Dino Workout: Low-Impact Moves for Maximum Longevity

Now, we know not everyone is looking to become the next velociraptor. Maybe you're more of a **lazy dino**, looking for low-impact moves that won't leave you sore and exhausted. Well, we've got you covered too.

The Low-Impact Advantage

Low-impact exercises are **gentle on your joints** and **easy on your body**. They're a great option for anyone with injuries, chronic pain, or just a preference for gentler workouts. Plus, they can be just as effective as high-impact exercises when it comes to improving your fitness and overall health.

Pro Tip: Incorporate low-impact exercises into your workout routine. Some good options include walking, swimming, cycling, and yoga. These exercises not only improve your fitness but also reduce stress, improve flexibility, and boost your mood.

The Yoga Yay

Yoga is a **fantastic** low-impact exercise that offers a **host of benefits**. It improves flexibility, strength, and balance, reduces stress, and even boosts your immune system. Plus, it's a great way to connect with your body and cultivate mindfulness.

Pro Tip: Find a yoga style that suits your needs and preferences. Some good options include Hatha yoga for beginners, Vinyasa yoga for a more dynamic practice, and Yin yoga for deep relaxation and flexibility.

The Pilates Power

Pilates is another **great** low-impact exercise that focuses on **core strength**, **posture**, and **alignment**. It's a fantastic way to improve your overall fitness, reduce back pain, and even enhance your athletic performance.

Pro Tip: Incorporate Pilates exercises into your workout routine. Some good options include the Hundred, the Roll-Up, the Single Leg Circle, and the Rolling Like a Ball. These exercises not only improve your core strength but also enhance your posture and flexibility.

The T-Rex Trot: Cardiovascular Exercise for Heart Health

Cardiovascular exercise is a **must** for anyone looking to improve their overall fitness and heart health. It gets your heart pumping, boosts your circulation, and even improves your mood. So, let's talk about how to **get your T-Rex trot on** and reap the benefits of cardiovascular exercise.

The Cardio Conundrum

Cardiovascular exercise, or **cardio** for short, is any exercise that **gets your heart rate up** and **keeps it there** for a sustained period. It's a great way to improve your heart health, boost your metabolism, and even reduce your risk of chronic diseases like heart disease and diabetes.

Pro Tip: Incorporate cardio exercises into your workout routine. Some good options include running, cycling, swimming, and dancing. Aim for **at least 30 minutes of moderate-intensity cardio most days of the week**.

The HIIT Hype

High-Intensity Interval Training, or **HIIT** for short, is a **type of cardio** that involves **short bursts of intense exercise** followed by **brief periods of rest**. It's a great way to boost your metabolism, improve your cardiovascular fitness, and even burn more calories in less time.

Pro Tip: Incorporate HIIT workouts into your workout routine. Some good options include Tabata workouts, which involve 20 seconds of intense exercise followed by 10 seconds of rest, repeated for 4 minutes. Or try a circuit workout, which involves moving from one exercise to the next with minimal rest in between.

The Steady-State Solution

Steady-state cardio is a **type of cardio** that involves **maintaining a consistent pace** for a sustained period. It's a great way to improve your endurance, reduce stress, and even enhance your mood. Plus, it's a fantastic option for anyone who prefers a more relaxed pace.

Pro Tip: Incorporate steady-state cardio into your workout routine. Some good options include jogging, cycling at a moderate pace, or swimming laps. Aim for **at least 30 minutes of steady-state cardio most days of the week**.

The Dino Dance: Flexibility and Mobility for Longevity

Flexibility and mobility are **crucial** for overall fitness and longevity. They help you move with ease, reduce your risk of injury, and even improve your posture. So, let's talk about how to **get your dino dance on** and reap the benefits of flexibility and mobility training.

The Flexibility Factor

Flexibility is all about **range of motion**. It's the ability to move your joints and muscles through their full range without pain or discomfort. And it's not just for yogis—flexibility is crucial for everyday life, from reaching for that top shelf to bending down to tie your shoes.

Pro Tip: Incorporate flexibility exercises into your workout routine. Some good options include static stretches, dynamic stretches, and foam rolling. Aim for **at least 10 minutes of stretching most days of the week**.

The Mobility Magic

Mobility is all about **functional movement**. It's the ability to move your body with ease and control, whether you're squatting down to pick up a heavy box or reaching up to grab a high branch. And it's a crucial component of overall fitness and longevity.

Pro Tip: Incorporate mobility exercises into your workout routine. Some good options include joint rotations, dynamic stretches, and animal flows. These exercises not only improve your mobility but also enhance your strength, balance, and coordination.

The Foam Rolling Fun

Foam rolling is a **great way** to improve your flexibility and mobility. It helps release tension, improve circulation, and even reduce pain and inflammation. Plus, it feels amazing—like a DIY massage for your muscles and fascia.

Pro Tip: Incorporate foam rolling into your workout routine. Focus on **tight spots** and **trigger points**, using slow, controlled movements to release tension and improve mobility. And don't forget to breathe—deep, steady breaths can help enhance the benefits of foam rolling.

The Balance Beam: Stability and Coordination for Everyday Life

Balance and coordination are **essential** for everyday life. They help you navigate uneven surfaces, catch yourself before a fall, and even improve your athletic performance. So, let's talk about how to **master the balance beam** and reap the benefits of stability and coordination training.

The Balance Benefit

Balance is all about **stability**. It's the ability to maintain your center of gravity over your base of support, whether you're standing on one leg or navigating a crowded sidewalk. And it's a crucial component of overall fitness and longevity.

Pro Tip: Incorporate balance exercises into your workout routine. Some good options include single-leg stands, heel-to-toe walks, and Tai Chi. Aim for **at least 10 minutes of balance training most days of the week**.

The Coordination Conundrum

Coordination is all about **timing** and **precision**. It's the ability to move your body with grace and control, whether you're dancing, playing a sport, or just walking down the street. And it's a crucial component of overall fitness and longevity.

Pro Tip: Incorporate coordination exercises into your workout routine. Some good options include jumping jacks, skipping, and agility drills. These exercises not only improve your coordination but also enhance your agility, strength, and cardiovascular fitness.

The Tai Chi Tranquility

Tai Chi is a **gentle, low-impact exercise** that combines **slow, flowing movements** with **deep, controlled breathing**. It's a fantastic way to improve your balance, coordination, and even your mental health. Plus, it's a great way to cultivate mindfulness and reduce stress.

Pro Tip: Incorporate Tai Chi into your workout routine. Look for a local class or follow along with an online video. And remember, Tai Chi is all about the journey, not the destination—so take your time, focus on your breath, and enjoy the process.

The Recovery Routine: Rest and Relaxation for Optimal Performance

Recovery is a **crucial** component of any fitness routine. It's the time when your body repairs and rebuilds, preparing you for your next workout. So, let's talk about how to **optimize your recovery** and reap the benefits of rest and relaxation.

The Sleep Solution

Sleep is **essential** for recovery. It's when your body produces growth hormones, repairs damaged tissues, and consolidates memories. Plus, it's a great way to reduce stress, improve your mood, and even enhance your cognitive function.

Pro Tip: Prioritize sleep. Aim for **7-9 hours of quality sleep per night**. Establish a relaxing bedtime routine, create a sleep sanctuary, and avoid screens before bed.

The Hydration Helper

Hydration is **crucial** for recovery. It helps transport nutrients, remove waste, and maintain the balance of electrolytes in your body. Plus, it's a key component of your cells' cytoplasm, the jelly-like substance that fills your cells.

Pro Tip: Stay hydrated. Aim for **eight 8-ounce glasses of water a day**. But remember, that's just a guideline. Your hydration needs can vary based on your activity level, climate, and overall health.

The Nutrition Nudge

Nutrition is a **big deal** when it comes to recovery. The right foods can help repair damaged tissues, reduce inflammation, and even enhance your immune function. Plus, they can provide the energy and nutrients you need to tackle your next workout.

Pro Tip: Focus on whole foods that are **rich in nutrients**. Some good options include fruits, vegetables, whole grains, lean proteins, and healthy fats. And don't forget to **time your meals**—eating within an hour of your workout can help optimize your recovery.

The Stretch and Soothe

Stretching and self-care are **essential** for recovery. They help release tension, improve circulation, and even reduce pain and inflammation. Plus, they can enhance your flexibility, mobility, and overall well-being.

Pro Tip: Incorporate stretching and self-care into your recovery routine. Some good options include static stretches, foam rolling, and massage. And don't forget to **listen to your body**—if something hurts, take a break and give your body the time it needs to heal.

The Mind-Body Connection: The Power of Mindfulness in Fitness

Mindfulness is a **powerful tool** when it comes to fitness. It can help you stay present, reduce stress, and even enhance your athletic performance. So, let's talk about how to **harness the power of mindfulness** and reap the benefits of the mind-body connection.

The Mindfulness Magic

Mindfulness is all about **being present**. It's the ability to focus on the here and now, without judgment or distraction. And it's a powerful tool for reducing stress, improving your mood, and even enhancing your cognitive function.

Pro Tip: Incorporate mindfulness practices into your fitness routine. Some good options include meditation, deep breathing, and body scan exercises. And remember, mindfulness is a skill—the more you practice, the better you get.

The Breathwork Benefit

Breathwork is a **great way** to cultivate mindfulness and enhance your fitness. It can help you stay present, reduce stress, and even improve your athletic performance. Plus, it's a fantastic way to connect with your body and cultivate a sense of calm and control.

Pro Tip: Incorporate breathwork exercises into your fitness routine. Some good options include box breathing, alternate nostril breathing, and the 4-7-8 technique. And remember, breathwork is all about the journey, not the destination—so take your time, focus on your breath, and enjoy the process.

The Visualization Victory

Visualization is a **powerful tool** for enhancing your athletic performance. It can help you stay focused, build confidence, and even improve your technique. Plus, it's a great way to cultivate mindfulness and reduce stress.

Pro Tip: Incorporate visualization exercises into your fitness routine. Imagine yourself performing at your best, visualize the movements and techniques you want to master, and focus on the feelings of success and accomplishment. And remember, visualization is a skill—the more you practice, the better you get.

The Fitness Formula: Putting It All Together

Now that we've talked about agility and strength training, low-impact exercises, cardiovascular exercise, flexibility and mobility, balance and coordination, recovery, and the mind-body connection, it's time to put it all together into a **fitness formula** that works for you.

The Customizable Workout

The key to a successful fitness routine is **customization**. What works for one person might not work for another, so it's important to find what works for you and make it a regular part of your routine.

Pro Tip: Create a customizable workout that includes exercises you enjoy and that fit your lifestyle and goals. Mix and match different types of exercises to keep things interesting and challenging. And don't forget to **listen to your body**—if something hurts, take a break and give your body the time it needs to heal.

The Fitness Schedule

Consistency is **key** when it comes to fitness. The more consistent you are, the better your results will be. So, it's important to create a **fitness schedule** that works for you and that you can stick to.

Pro Tip: Create a fitness schedule that includes a mix of different types of exercises. Aim for **at least 30 minutes of exercise most days of the week**, with a mix of strength training, cardio, flexibility, and balance exercises. And don't forget to **schedule rest days**—your body needs time to recover and rebuild.

The Accountability Factor

Accountability is a **big deal** when it comes to fitness. It can help you stay motivated, track your progress, and even enhance your results. So, it's important to find ways to **hold yourself accountable** and stay on track.

Pro Tip: Find an accountability partner—someone who shares your fitness goals and can help keep you motivated and on track. Or use a **fitness tracker** or **app** to track your progress and stay accountable. And don't forget to **celebrate your successes**—whether it's hitting a new personal best or just sticking to your fitness routine, every victory is worth celebrating.

CHAPTER 6: STRESS MANAGEMENT: TAMING YOUR INNER T-REX

Alright, folks! We've talked about diet, exercise, and all the good stuff that keeps your inner dinosaur roaring. But now it's time to tackle a **major** culprit that can wreak havoc on your cells: **stress**. Think of this chapter as your ultimate guide to **taming your inner T-Rex** and keeping your stress levels in check.

The Fight or Flight Response: Your Body's Ancient Alarm System

Before we dive into stress management, let's talk about the **fight or flight response**. This is your body's **ancient alarm system**, designed to help you deal with immediate threats. But in today's world, it can often do more harm than good.

The Stress Response Explained

When you're stressed, your body goes into **fight or flight mode**. Your heart rate increases, your blood pressure goes up, and your body pumps out stress hormones like **cortisol** and **adrenaline**. This response is great for dealing with short-term threats, like, say, a hungry T-Rex. But when it's constantly activated, it can lead to a host of health issues.

Fun Fact: The fight or flight response is controlled by the **sympathetic nervous system**, which is responsible for regulating your body's involuntary functions, like heart rate and digestion.

The Chronic Stress Conundrum

Chronic stress is a **big deal**. It can lead to everything from high blood pressure to weakened immunity to accelerated aging. Plus, it can wreak havoc on your mental health, leading to anxiety, depression, and even burnout.

Pro Tip: Recognize the signs of chronic stress. Some common symptoms include fatigue, irritability, headaches, digestive issues, and sleep disturbances. If you're experiencing any of these symptoms, it might be time to take a closer look at your stress levels.

The Inflammation Connection: How Stress Affects Your Cells

Stress doesn't just affect your mental health—it also takes a toll on your cells. One of the ways it does this is through **inflammation**.

The Inflammation Lowdown

Inflammation is your body's response to injury or infection. It's a good thing when it's acute (short-term), but chronic (long-term) inflammation can wreak havoc on your cells, leading to everything from wrinkles to heart disease.

Pro Tip: Reduce inflammation by **managing stress**. Practices like mindfulness, exercise, and a healthy diet can all help reduce inflammation and keep your cells happy and healthy.

The Cortisol Crisis

Cortisol is a **stress hormone** that plays a crucial role in your body's fight or flight response. But when it's constantly elevated, it can lead to a host of health issues, including inflammation, weakened immunity, and even weight gain.

Pro Tip: Manage cortisol levels by **practicing stress-reducing techniques**. Some good options include deep breathing, meditation, and progressive muscle relaxation.

The Mind-Body Connection: The Power of Mindfulness

Mindfulness is a **powerful tool** when it comes to stress management. It can help you stay present, reduce stress, and even enhance your overall well-being. So, let's talk about how to **harness the power of mindfulness** and reap the benefits of the mind-body connection.

The Mindfulness Magic

Mindfulness is all about **being present**. It's the ability to focus on the here and now, without judgment or distraction. And it's a powerful tool for reducing stress, improving your mood, and even enhancing your cognitive function.

Pro Tip: Incorporate mindfulness practices into your daily routine. Some good options include meditation, deep breathing, and body scan exercises. And remember, mindfulness is a skill—the more you practice, the better you get.

The Meditation Miracle

Meditation is a **fantastic** way to cultivate mindfulness and reduce stress. It can help you stay present, calm your mind, and even improve your overall health. Plus, it's a great way to connect with your body and cultivate a sense of peace and tranquility.

Pro Tip: Find a meditation style that suits your needs and preferences. Some good options include mindfulness meditation, loving-kindness meditation, and transcendental meditation. And remember, meditation is all about the journey, not the destination—so take your time, focus on your breath, and enjoy the process.

The Breathwork Benefit

Breathwork is a **great way** to cultivate mindfulness and reduce stress. It can help you stay present, calm your mind, and even improve your overall health. Plus, it's a fantastic way to connect with your body and cultivate a sense of calm and control.

Pro Tip: Incorporate breathwork exercises into your daily routine. Some good options include box breathing, alternate nostril breathing, and the 4-7-8 technique. And remember, breathwork is all about the journey, not the destination—so take your time, focus on your breath, and enjoy the process.

The Exercise Effect: How Movement Reduces Stress

Exercise is a **powerful tool** when it comes to stress management. It can help reduce stress hormones, increase the production of endorphins (your body's natural mood boosters), and even improve your overall health. So, let's talk about how to **harness the power of exercise** and reap the benefits of movement.

The Endorphin Rush

Endorphins are **natural mood boosters** that your body produces in response to exercise. They can help reduce stress, improve your mood, and even enhance your overall well-being. Plus, they can make exercise feel more enjoyable, which can help keep you motivated and on track.

Pro Tip: Find an exercise you enjoy and make it a regular part of your routine. Whether it's running, cycling, swimming, or dancing, the key is to find something that brings you joy and makes you want to move.

The Cardio Calm

Cardiovascular exercise is a **great way** to reduce stress and improve your overall health. It gets your heart pumping, boosts your circulation, and even improves your mood. Plus, it can help reduce stress hormones and increase the production of endorphins.

Pro Tip: Incorporate cardio exercises into your workout routine. Some good options include running, cycling, swimming, and dancing. Aim for **at least 30 minutes of moderate-intensity cardio most days of the week**.

The Strength Solution

Strength training is another **great way** to reduce stress and improve your overall health. It helps build and maintain muscle mass, boosts your metabolism, and even improves your bone density. Plus, it can help reduce stress hormones and increase the production of endorphins.

Pro Tip: Focus on compound movements that work multiple muscle groups at once. Some good options include squats, deadlifts, lunges, push-ups, and pull-ups. And remember, you don't need a fancy gym membership to get strong—bodyweight exercises and simple equipment like dumbbells and resistance bands can be just as effective.

The Social Support System: The Power of Connection

Social support is a **crucial** component of stress management. It can help buffer the effects of stress, improve your overall well-being, and even enhance your resilience. So, let's talk about how to **harness the power of connection** and reap the benefits of social support.

The Connection Conundrum

Connection is a **basic human need**. It's the feeling of being seen, heard, and valued by others. And it's a crucial component of overall well-being and resilience. But in today's fast-paced, always-connected world, it can be easy to feel disconnected and isolated.

Pro Tip: Prioritize connection. Make time for the people who matter most to you, whether it's family, friends, or even your furry companions. And don't be afraid to reach out and ask for help when you need it—we all need a little support sometimes.

The Support Squad

Your support squad is the **group of people** who have your back, no matter what. They're the ones you can turn to for advice, comfort, and encouragement. And they're a crucial component of stress management and overall well-being.

Pro Tip: Build your support squad. Surround yourself with people who uplift and inspire you, who listen and understand you, and who support and encourage you. And remember, quality is more important than quantity—it's better to have a few close friends than a hundred acquaintances.

The Community Connection

Community is a **powerful force** when it comes to stress management and overall well-being. It can provide a sense of belonging, purpose, and connection. Plus, it can offer opportunities for support, encouragement, and even collaboration.

Pro Tip: Get involved in your community. Join a club or group that aligns with your interests and values. Volunteer for a cause you care about. Or simply connect with your neighbors and build a sense of community where you live. And remember, community is all about give and take—the more you put in, the more you get out.

The Sleep Solution: The Power of Rest and Recovery

Sleep is **essential** for stress management and overall well-being. It's when your body repairs and rebuilds, preparing you for the challenges of the day ahead. So, let's talk about how to **harness the power of sleep** and reap the benefits of rest and recovery.

The Sleep-Stress Connection

Sleep and stress are **closely linked**. When you're stressed, it can be hard to fall asleep and stay asleep. And when you're not getting enough sleep, it can exacerbate the effects of stress, leading to a vicious cycle of sleepless nights and stressful days.

Pro Tip: Prioritize sleep. Aim for **7-9 hours of quality sleep per night**. Establish a relaxing bedtime routine, create a sleep sanctuary, and avoid screens before bed.

The Relaxation Routine

Relaxation is a **crucial** component of stress management and overall well-being. It can help calm your mind, reduce stress hormones, and even improve your sleep quality. So, let's talk about how to **incorporate relaxation** into your daily routine.

Pro Tip: Establish a relaxation routine. Some good options include deep breathing, progressive muscle relaxation, and guided imagery. And remember, relaxation is all about finding what works for you—whether it's a warm bath, a good book, or a quiet moment of reflection, the key is to find what brings you peace and makes you feel calm and centered.

The Power Nap

Napping is a **great way** to recharge and rejuvenate, especially when you're feeling stressed or overwhelmed. It can help improve your mood, boost your energy, and even enhance your cognitive function. Plus, it can be a fantastic way to catch up on missed sleep and reduce the effects of sleep deprivation.

Pro Tip: Take a power nap. Aim for **20-30 minutes** of uninterrupted sleep, preferably in a quiet, dark, and comfortable environment. And remember, the key to a successful power nap is to set an alarm—you don't want to oversleep and wake up feeling groggy and disoriented.

The Nutrition Nudge: The Power of Food

Nutrition is a **big deal** when it comes to stress management and overall well-being. The right foods can help reduce stress, improve your mood, and even enhance your cognitive function. So, let's talk about how to **harness the power of food** and reap the benefits of good nutrition.

The Stress-Busting Diet

A stress-busting diet is all about **nourishing your body** and **calming your mind**. It's packed with nutrient-dense foods that support your overall health and well-being, while also helping to reduce stress and improve your mood.

Pro Tip: Focus on whole foods that are **rich in nutrients**. Some good options include fruits, vegetables, whole grains, lean proteins, and healthy fats. And don't forget to **stay hydrated**—dehydration can exacerbate the effects of stress and lead to a host of other health issues.

The Magnesium Magic

Magnesium is a **mineral** that plays a crucial role in stress management and overall well-being. It helps regulate nerve and muscle function, supports a healthy immune system, and even promotes relaxation and sleep. Plus, it can help reduce stress, improve your mood, and even enhance your cognitive function.

Pro Tip: Incorporate magnesium-rich foods into your diet. Some good options include leafy greens, nuts, seeds, and whole grains. And if you're not getting enough magnesium through your diet, consider supplementing with a high-quality magnesium supplement.

The Omega-3 Advantage

Omega-3 fatty acids are **essential fats** that play a crucial role in stress management and overall well-being. They help reduce inflammation, support a healthy immune system, and even improve your mood and cognitive function. Plus, they can help reduce stress, improve your sleep quality, and even enhance your overall health.

Pro Tip: Incorporate omega-3-rich foods into your diet. Some good options include fatty fish like salmon and mackerel, walnuts, chia seeds, and flaxseeds. And if you're not getting enough omega-3s through your diet, consider supplementing with a high-quality fish oil or algae-based supplement.

The Time Management Trick: The Power of Prioritization

Time management is a **crucial** component of stress management and overall well-being. It can help you stay organized, reduce overwhelm, and even enhance your productivity. So, let's talk about how to **harness the power of prioritization** and reap the benefits of effective time management.

The Prioritization Puzzle

Prioritization is all about **focusing on what matters most**. It's the ability to identify your most important tasks and allocate your time and energy accordingly. And it's a crucial component of stress management and overall well-being.

Pro Tip: Use the Eisenhower Matrix to **prioritize your tasks**. This simple tool helps you categorize your tasks based on their urgency and importance, allowing you to focus on what matters most and eliminate the rest.

The To-Do List Tactic

A to-do list is a **powerful tool** when it comes to time management and stress reduction. It can help you stay organized, reduce overwhelm, and even enhance your productivity. Plus, it can provide a sense of accomplishment and satisfaction as you cross off each task.

Pro Tip: Create a to-do list that includes your most important tasks for the day. Break down larger tasks into smaller, manageable steps, and prioritize based on urgency and importance. And don't forget to **celebrate your successes**—whether it's completing a task or simply making progress, every victory is worth celebrating.

The Boundary Battle

Boundaries are a **crucial** component of time management and stress reduction. They help you protect your time and energy, reduce overwhelm, and even enhance your overall well-being. Plus, they can provide a sense of control and empowerment, allowing you to take charge of your life and prioritize what matters most.

Pro Tip: Set boundaries around your time and energy. Learn to say no to tasks and commitments that don't align with your priorities and values. And don't be afraid to **delegate**—whether it's asking for help with a task or outsourcing a responsibility, delegation can be a powerful tool for reducing stress and enhancing productivity.

The Mindset Makeover: The Power of Positive Thinking

Mindset is a **powerful force** when it comes to stress management and overall well-being. It can help you stay resilient, reduce stress, and even enhance your overall health. So, let's talk about how to **harness the power of positive thinking** and reap the benefits of a mindset makeover.

The Positivity Principle

Positivity is all about **focusing on the good**. It's the ability to see the silver lining in every cloud, to find the opportunity in every challenge, and to cultivate a sense of gratitude and appreciation for the blessings in your life. And it's a powerful tool for reducing stress, improving your mood, and even enhancing your overall health.

Pro Tip: Cultivate a positive mindset by **focusing on the good** in your life. Practice gratitude, surround yourself with positive people, and engage in activities that bring you joy and fulfillment. And remember, positivity is a skill—the more you practice, the better you get.

The Gratitude Gambit

Gratitude is a **powerful practice** when it comes to stress management and overall well-being. It can help you stay present, reduce stress, and even enhance your overall health. Plus, it can provide a sense of perspective and appreciation, allowing you to see the blessings in your life and cultivate a sense of contentment and satisfaction.

Pro Tip: Practice gratitude by **keeping a gratitude journal**. Each day, write down three things you're grateful for, no matter how big or small. And don't forget to **express your gratitude**—whether it's thanking a friend for their support or acknowledging a colleague for their hard work, expressing gratitude can strengthen your relationships and enhance your overall well-being.

The Reframing Routine

Reframing is a **powerful tool** when it comes to stress management and overall well-being. It's the ability to see challenges and setbacks as opportunities for growth and learning, rather than as threats or failures. And it's a crucial component of resilience and overall well-being.

Pro Tip: Practice reframing by **looking for the opportunity** in every challenge. Ask yourself, "What can I learn from this experience? How can I grow and improve as a result of this challenge?" And remember, reframing is a skill—the more you practice, the better you get.

CHAPTER 7: THE DINO DOC'S GUIDE TO MODERN MEDICINE

Alright, folks! We've talked about diet, exercise, stress management, and all the good stuff that keeps your inner dinosaur roaring. But now it's time to dive into the world of **modern medicine**. Think of this chapter as your ultimate guide to navigating the healthcare jungle and making the most of your doctor visits.

Navigating the Healthcare Jungle: Tips and Tricks

The healthcare system can be a **confusing and overwhelming** place. But with the right tools and strategies, you can navigate it like a pro. So, let's talk about how to **make the most of your healthcare experience**.

The Doctor-Patient Relationship: Building Trust and Communication

The relationship between you and your doctor is **crucial** for your overall health and well-being. It's built on trust, communication, and mutual respect. So, let's talk about how to **build a strong and effective doctor-patient relationship**.

Pro Tip: Find a doctor you trust. Look for someone who listens to your concerns, answers your questions, and involves you in decision-making. A good doctor-patient relationship is built on open communication and mutual respect.

The Art of Asking Questions: Getting the Answers You Need

Asking the right questions is **key** to getting the information you need from your doctor. But it's not always easy to know what to ask or how to ask it. So, let's talk about the **art of asking questions** and getting the answers you need.

Pro Tip: Prepare a list of questions before your appointment. Write down any concerns, symptoms, or questions you have, and bring the list with you to your appointment. This will help you stay organized and ensure that you get all the information you need.

The Power of Advocacy: Standing Up for Your Health

Advocating for yourself is **crucial** when it comes to your health. It means speaking up, asking questions, and making sure your needs are met. So, let's talk about the **power of advocacy** and how to **stand up for your health**.

Pro Tip: Be your own advocate. Don't be afraid to speak up, ask questions, and make sure your needs are met. Remember, you are the expert on your own body, and your input is valuable.

The Preventive Care Plan: Staying Ahead of the Game

Preventive care is all about **staying ahead of the game**. It's about catching health issues early, before they become major problems. So, let's talk about the **preventive care plan** and how to **keep your health on track**.

The Annual Check-Up: Your Healthcare Maintenance Plan

Annual check-ups are a **key component** of preventive care. They give you and your doctor a chance to review your health, catch any issues early, and make a plan for the future. So, let's talk about the **annual check-up** and how to **make the most of it**.

Pro Tip: Schedule an annual check-up with your doctor. Use this time to review your health, discuss any concerns, and make a plan for the future. And don't forget to **follow up** on any tests or referrals your doctor recommends.

The Screenings and Tests: Catching Issues Early

Screenings and tests are a **crucial part** of preventive care. They help catch health issues early, before they become major problems. So, let's talk about the **screenings and tests** you need and how to **stay on top of them**.

Pro Tip: Stay up-to-date on your screenings and tests. Talk to your doctor about which screenings are right for you, based on your age, gender, and health history. And don't forget to **follow up** on any abnormal results.

The Vaccination Station: Protecting Your Health

Vaccinations are a **key component** of preventive care. They help protect you from a variety of diseases and keep you healthy. So, let's talk about the **vaccination station** and how to **stay up-to-date** on your shots.

Pro Tip: Stay up-to-date on your vaccinations. Talk to your doctor about which vaccines are right for you, based on your age, health history, and lifestyle. And don't forget to **follow up** on any booster shots or additional vaccines you may need.

The Chronic Condition Conundrum: Managing Long-Term Health Issues

Chronic conditions are a **major challenge** for many people. They require ongoing management, monitoring, and care. So, let's talk about the **chronic condition conundrum** and how to **manage long-term health issues**.

The Management Plan: Staying on Top of Your Health

Managing a chronic condition requires a **comprehensive plan**. It involves regular check-ups, medication management, lifestyle changes, and more. So, let's talk about the **management plan** and how to **stay on top of your health**.

Pro Tip: Work with your doctor to create a **management plan** for your chronic condition. This plan should include regular check-ups, medication management, lifestyle changes, and any other treatments or therapies you need.

The Medication Maze: Navigating Your Prescriptions

Medications are a **key component** of managing chronic conditions. But they can also be confusing and overwhelming. So, let's talk about the **medication maze** and how to **navigate your prescriptions**.

Pro Tip: Keep a list of your medications, including the name, dose, and frequency. Bring this list with you to your appointments, and make sure your doctor is aware of all the medications you're taking. And don't forget to **ask questions** about any new medications or changes to your regimen.

The Lifestyle Changes: Making Healthy Choices

Lifestyle changes are a **crucial part** of managing chronic conditions. They can help improve your symptoms, reduce your risk of complications, and even enhance your overall health. So, let's talk about the **lifestyle changes** you need to make and how to **stick to them**.

Pro Tip: Make healthy choices that support your overall health and well-being. This might include changes to your diet, exercise routine, sleep habits, and more. And don't forget to **set realistic goals** and **track your progress**—celebrating your successes along the way.

The Emergency Room Etiquette: What to Do in a Crisis

Emergencies happen, and when they do, it's important to know what to do. So, let's talk about **emergency room etiquette** and how to **handle a crisis** like a pro.

The ER Visit: What to Expect and How to Prepare

Visiting the emergency room can be a **stressful and overwhelming** experience. But knowing what to expect and how to prepare can make all the difference. So, let's talk about the **ER visit** and how to **make the most of it**.

Pro Tip: Prepare for your ER visit by bringing a list of your medications, any relevant medical records, and a trusted friend or family member. And don't forget to **stay calm** and **communicate clearly** with the medical staff—they're there to help you.

The Follow-Up Care: Continuing Your Recovery

After an emergency room visit, it's important to **follow up** with your doctor and continue your recovery. So, let's talk about the **follow-up care** and how to **stay on track**.

Pro Tip: Schedule a follow-up appointment with your doctor after your ER visit. Use this time to review your diagnosis, discuss any follow-up tests or treatments, and make a plan for your recovery. And don't forget to **follow your doctor's instructions**—they're there to help you heal and get back on your feet.

The Mental Health Matters: Caring for Your Mind and Body

Mental health is a **crucial component** of overall health and well-being. It affects how you think, feel, and act, and it can have a **major impact** on your physical health. So, let's talk about **mental health matters** and how to **care for your mind and body**.

The Mental Health Check-Up: Assessing Your Well-Being

Just like your physical health, your mental health needs **regular check-ups**. So, let's talk about the **mental health check-up** and how to **assess your well-being**.

Pro Tip: Schedule a mental health check-up with your doctor. Use this time to discuss any concerns, symptoms, or challenges you're facing. And don't forget to **be honest**—your doctor is there to help you, not judge you.

The Therapy Talk: Finding the Right Support

Therapy is a **powerful tool** for managing mental health issues. It can help you process your emotions, develop coping strategies, and even enhance your overall well-being. So, let's talk about the **therapy talk** and how to **find the right support**.

Pro Tip: Find a therapist who is a **good fit** for you. Look for someone who specializes in the issues you're facing, who listens to your concerns, and who makes you feel comfortable and supported. And don't forget to **shop around**—it's okay to try out a few different therapists before finding the right one.

The Self-Care Strategy: Nurturing Your Mind and Body

Self-care is a **crucial component** of mental health and overall well-being. It involves taking care of your physical, emotional, and mental needs. So, let's talk about the **self-care strategy** and how to **nurture your mind and body**.

Pro Tip: Practice self-care by engaging in activities that **nurture your mind and body**. This might include exercise, meditation, journaling, spending time in nature, or simply taking a moment to relax and unwind. And remember, self-care is not selfish—it's essential for your overall health and well-being.

The Insurance Ins and Outs: Navigating Your Coverage

Health insurance can be a **confusing and overwhelming** topic. But understanding your coverage is **crucial** for making informed decisions about your healthcare. So, let's talk about the **insurance ins and outs** and how to **navigate your coverage**.

The Coverage Conundrum: Understanding Your Plan

Understanding your health insurance plan is **key** to making informed decisions about your healthcare. So, let's talk about the **coverage conundrum** and how to **understand your plan**.

Pro Tip: Review your health insurance plan carefully. Make sure you understand what's covered, what's not, and any out-of-pocket costs you might be responsible for. And don't be afraid to **ask questions**—your insurance provider is there to help you.

The Claims Process: Getting the Care You Need

Filing a claim can be a **daunting** task. But knowing how to navigate the claims process can make all the difference. So, let's talk about the **claims process** and how to **get the care you need**.

Pro Tip: Keep detailed records of all your medical appointments, tests, and treatments. This will help you when it comes time to file a claim. And don't forget to **follow up**— if you don't hear back about your claim, don't be afraid to reach out and ask for an update.

The Appeals Process: Fighting for Your Rights

Sometimes, insurance companies make **mistakes** or **deny claims** that should be covered. When this happens, it's important to know your rights and how to **fight for the care you need**. So, let's talk about the **appeals process** and how to **advocate for yourself**.

Pro Tip: Know your rights and **don't be afraid to appeal** a denied claim. Gather all the necessary documentation, follow the appeals process outlined by your insurance provider, and don't be afraid to **seek help** from a patient advocate or legal professional if needed.

The Alternative Medicine Approach: Exploring Other Options

Alternative medicine offers a **range of options** for those looking to complement or supplement their traditional healthcare. So, let's talk about the **alternative medicine approach** and how to **explore other options**.

The Complementary Care: Integrating Different Approaches

Complementary care involves **integrating** different approaches to healthcare. It can include everything from acupuncture to chiropractic care to herbal remedies. So, let's talk about **complementary care** and how to **integrate different approaches**.

Pro Tip: Talk to your doctor about any complementary care approaches you're considering. Make sure they're aware of any supplements, treatments, or therapies you're using, and discuss how they might fit into your overall healthcare plan.

The Holistic Health: Treating the Whole Person

Holistic health is all about **treating the whole person**. It considers the physical, emotional, mental, and spiritual aspects of health and well-being. So, let's talk about **holistic health** and how to **treat the whole person**.

Pro Tip: Find a holistic healthcare provider who takes a **whole-person approach** to your health. Look for someone who considers your physical, emotional, mental, and spiritual needs, and who involves you in decision-making.

The Natural Remedies: Harnessing the Power of Nature

Natural remedies offer a **range of options** for those looking to complement or supplement their traditional healthcare. So, let's talk about **natural remedies** and how to **harness the power of nature.**

Pro Tip: Do your research before trying any natural remedies. Make sure they're safe, effective, and appropriate for your needs. And don't forget to **talk to your doctor**—they can help you understand the potential benefits and risks of any natural remedies you're considering.

CHAPTER 8: DINO-PROOFING YOUR ENVIRONMENT: HOME SWEET HABITAT

Alright, folks! We've talked about diet, exercise, stress management, and navigating the healthcare jungle. Now it's time to dive into the world of **environmental health**. Think of this chapter as your ultimate guide to **dino-proofing your environment** and creating a **home sweet habitat** that supports your overall health and well-being.

The Air You Breathe: Creating a Clean and Healthy Atmosphere

The air you breathe is a **major factor** in your overall health and well-being. But unfortunately, our modern world is full of pollutants, allergens, and other irritants that can wreak havoc on your respiratory system. So, let's talk about how to **create a clean and healthy atmosphere** in your home.

The Indoor Air Quality Quandary

Indoor air quality is a **big deal**. It can affect everything from your respiratory health to your cognitive function. But unfortunately, many of our homes are filled with pollutants, allergens, and other irritants that can compromise our health.

Pro Tip: Invest in an air purifier for your home. Look for one with a HEPA filter, which can remove up to 99.97% of airborne particles. Also, consider adding some **houseplants** to your space. Plants like snake plants, spider plants, and peace lilies are known for their air-purifying properties.

The Ventilation Vibe

Proper ventilation is **crucial** for maintaining good indoor air quality. It helps remove pollutants, allergens, and other irritants from your home, keeping the air fresh and clean.

Pro Tip: Open your windows regularly to allow fresh air to circulate. Also, consider installing a **ventilation system** in your home, especially in areas like the kitchen and bathroom, where moisture and odors can build up.

The Dust and Dander Dilemma

Dust and dander are **common allergens** that can trigger a variety of respiratory issues, from sneezing and coughing to asthma attacks. But with the right strategies, you can keep these irritants at bay and maintain a clean and healthy atmosphere in your home.

Pro Tip: Dust and vacuum your home regularly to remove dust and dander. Use a vacuum with a HEPA filter to trap allergens, and consider using a **damp cloth** to dust surfaces, which can help prevent dust from becoming airborne.

The Water You Drink: Ensuring Pure and Safe Hydration

Water is **essential** for your overall health and well-being. It helps transport nutrients, remove waste, and maintain the balance of electrolytes in your body. But not all water is created equal. So, let's talk about how to **ensure pure and safe hydration** in your home.

The Water Quality Conundrum

Water quality is a **major concern** for many people. Tap water can contain a variety of contaminants, from chlorine and lead to even pharmaceutical residues. But with the right strategies, you can ensure that the water you drink is pure and safe.

Pro Tip: Invest in a water filter for your home. Look for one that's certified by the National Sanitation Foundation (NSF) to remove a wide range of contaminants. Also, consider using a **reusable water bottle** to reduce your exposure to plastic chemicals and minimize your environmental impact.

The Bottled Water Blues

Bottled water is a **convenient** option, but it's not always the best choice for your health or the environment. Many bottled waters are simply filtered tap water, and the plastic bottles can leach harmful chemicals into the water, especially when heated.

Pro Tip: Avoid bottled water whenever possible. Instead, opt for filtered tap water and use a reusable water bottle. And if you do choose to drink bottled water, look for brands that use BPA-free bottles and have a good track record for water quality.

The Hydration Habit

Staying hydrated is **crucial** for your overall health and well-being. It helps maintain your body's fluid balance, supports your digestive system, and even enhances your cognitive function.

Pro Tip: Aim for eight 8-ounce glasses of water a day. But remember, that's just a guideline. Your hydration needs can vary based on your activity level, climate, and overall health. And don't forget to **listen to your body**—if you're feeling thirsty, it's a sign that you need to hydrate.

The Products You Use: Choosing Safe and Natural Options

The products you use in your home can have a **major impact** on your health and well-being. From cleaning supplies to personal care products, many of these items contain chemicals that can be harmful to your health. So, let's talk about how to **choose safe and natural options** for your home.

The Cleaning Conundrum

Cleaning products are a **necessary evil** in our modern world. They help keep our homes clean and free of germs, but many of them contain harsh chemicals that can be harmful to our health.

Pro Tip: Opt for natural and organic cleaning products whenever possible. Look for products that are free from parabens, phthalates, sulfates, and other harmful chemicals. Also, consider making your own cleaning products using natural ingredients like vinegar, baking soda, and essential oils.

The Personal Care Puzzle

Personal care products are a **big part** of our daily routines. But many of these products contain chemicals that can be harmful to our health, from endocrine disruptors to carcinogens.

Pro Tip: Choose natural and organic personal care products whenever possible. Look for products that are free from parabens, phthalates, sulfates, and other harmful chemicals. Also, consider making your own personal care products using natural ingredients like coconut oil, shea butter, and essential oils.

The Fragrance Factor

Fragrances are a **common ingredient** in many household and personal care products. But many of these fragrances contain chemicals that can be harmful to our health, from endocrine disruptors to respiratory irritants.

Pro Tip: Avoid products with synthetic fragrances. Instead, opt for products that are fragrance-free or scented with natural essential oils. And if you do choose to use fragranced products, look for brands that use natural and organic ingredients and have a good track record for safety.

The Radiation Rundown: Minimizing Your Exposure

Radiation is a **fact of life**. It comes from the sun, the earth, and even the food we eat. But while a little bit of radiation is unavoidable, too much can be harmful. So, let's talk about how to **minimize your exposure** to radiation in your home.

The Electromagnetic Radiation Enigma

Electromagnetic radiation is a **type of radiation** that comes from electronic devices like cell phones, computers, and Wi-Fi routers. While the jury is still out on the long-term effects of this type of radiation, many experts recommend taking steps to minimize your exposure.

Pro Tip: Limit your exposure to electromagnetic radiation by turning off your devices when you're not using them, using a landline for long phone calls, and keeping your devices away from your body whenever possible.

The UV Radiation Reality

UV radiation is a **type of radiation** that comes from the sun. While a little bit of sun exposure is necessary for vitamin D production, too much can be harmful, leading to everything from sunburn to skin cancer.

Pro Tip: Protect yourself from UV radiation by wearing sunscreen, protective clothing, and a hat when you're out in the sun. Also, consider staying in the shade during peak sun hours, typically between 10 am and 4 pm.

The Radon Risk

Radon is a **naturally occurring radioactive gas** that can seep into homes through cracks in the foundation, walls, and floors. It's a leading cause of lung cancer in the United States, and it's a major concern for many homeowners.

Pro Tip: Test your home for radon using a radon test kit, which you can purchase at most hardware stores or online. If your home tests positive for radon, consider hiring a professional to install a radon mitigation system.

The Mold and Mildew Mystery: Keeping Your Home Dry and Clean

Mold and mildew are **common issues** in many homes. They can cause a variety of health problems, from respiratory issues to allergic reactions. But with the right strategies, you can keep your home dry and clean and prevent mold and mildew from taking hold.

The Moisture Management Plan

Managing moisture is **key** to preventing mold and mildew in your home. It involves controlling humidity levels, fixing leaks, and ensuring proper ventilation.

Pro Tip: Control humidity levels in your home by using a dehumidifier, especially in areas like the basement, bathroom, and kitchen. Also, **fix any leaks** promptly to prevent moisture from building up, and **ensure proper ventilation** by opening windows and using exhaust fans.

The Cleaning and Maintenance Routine

Regular cleaning and maintenance are **crucial** for preventing mold and mildew in your home. It involves cleaning surfaces, inspecting for signs of mold, and addressing any issues promptly.

Pro Tip: Clean surfaces regularly using a solution of water and vinegar, which can help kill mold and mildew. Also, **inspect your home** for signs of mold, such as musty odors, water stains, or visible mold growth. And if you do find mold, **address it promptly** by cleaning the affected area and fixing any underlying moisture issues.

The Professional Help Option

Sometimes, mold and mildew issues are too big to handle on your own. In these cases, it's important to **seek professional help** to ensure that the problem is addressed properly and safely.

Pro Tip: Hire a professional mold remediation company if you have a significant mold problem in your home. Look for a company that is licensed, insured, and has a good track record for safety and effectiveness. And don't forget to **follow up** with any recommended repairs or maintenance to prevent future mold issues.

The Pest Control Plan: Keeping Unwanted Guests at Bay

Pests are a **common problem** in many homes. They can cause a variety of issues, from property damage to health problems. But with the right strategies, you can keep unwanted guests at bay and maintain a pest-free home.

The Prevention Plan

Prevention is **key** to keeping pests out of your home. It involves sealing entry points, maintaining a clean and clutter-free environment, and addressing any moisture issues promptly.

Pro Tip: Seal entry points in your home, such as cracks, gaps, and holes, using caulk, weatherstripping, or other sealants. Also, **maintain a clean and clutter-free environment** by regularly cleaning surfaces, removing food sources, and addressing any moisture issues promptly.

The Natural Repellents Option

Natural repellents are a **great option** for keeping pests at bay without the use of harsh chemicals. They can be just as effective as chemical repellents, and they're safer for your health and the environment.

Pro Tip: Use natural repellents like essential oils, diatomaceous earth, and borax to keep pests at bay. Also, consider using **physical barriers** like screens, nets, and traps to prevent pests from entering your home.

The Professional Help Option

Sometimes, pest issues are too big to handle on your own. In these cases, it's important to **seek professional help** to ensure that the problem is addressed properly and safely.

Pro Tip: Hire a professional pest control company if you have a significant pest problem in your home. Look for a company that is licensed, insured, and has a good track record for safety and effectiveness. And don't forget to **follow up** with any recommended repairs or maintenance to prevent future pest issues.

The Green Thumb Guide: Cultivating a Healthy Indoor Environment

Plants are a **great way** to enhance the indoor environment of your home. They can improve air quality, reduce stress, and even boost your mood. So, let's talk about how to **cultivate a healthy indoor environment** with the help of plants.

The Air-Purifying Powerhouses

Certain plants are **known for their air-purifying properties**. They can help remove pollutants, allergens, and other irritants from the air, improving the overall air quality in your home.

Pro Tip: Choose air-purifying plants like snake plants, spider plants, and peace lilies for your home. These plants are known for their ability to remove a variety of pollutants from the air, including formaldehyde, benzene, and trichloroethylene.

The Stress-Reducing Benefits

Plants are a **great way** to reduce stress and enhance your overall well-being. They can provide a sense of calm and tranquility, and they can even boost your mood and cognitive function.

Pro Tip: Place plants in areas of your home where you spend a lot of time, such as your living room, bedroom, and office. Also, consider choosing plants that are **easy to care for** and **low-maintenance**, so you can enjoy their benefits without a lot of effort.

The Aesthetic Appeal

Plants are a **great way** to enhance the aesthetic appeal of your home. They can add a touch of nature, color, and texture to your space, making it feel more inviting and comfortable.

Pro Tip: Choose plants that complement the style and decor of your home. Also, consider grouping plants together to create a **lush and vibrant** display, or using them to **soften hard edges** and **add warmth** to your space.

CHAPTER 9: THE SOCIAL DINOSAUR: BUILDING YOUR PREHISTORIC POSSE

Alright, folks! We've talked about diet, exercise, stress management, and creating a healthy home environment. Now it's time to dive into the world of **social health**. Think of this chapter as your ultimate guide to **building your prehistoric posse** and creating a supportive social network that enhances your overall health and well-being.

The Power of Connection: Why Social Health Matters

Social health is a **crucial component** of overall well-being. It's about the quality of your relationships, the strength of your social network, and the sense of belonging and connection you feel with others. So, let's talk about why **social health matters** and how to **build a strong and supportive social network**.

The Loneliness Epidemic: The Impact of Social Isolation

Loneliness is a **major public health issue** in today's world. It can lead to a host of health problems, from depression and anxiety to heart disease and even a weakened immune system. But the good news is, there are steps you can take to combat loneliness and build a strong and supportive social network.

Pro Tip: Recognize the signs of loneliness. If you're feeling isolated, disconnected, or like you don't have anyone to turn to, it might be time to reach out and build some new connections.

The Support System: The Importance of Strong Relationships

Strong relationships are the **backbone** of social health. They provide a sense of belonging, support, and connection that can enhance your overall well-being and resilience. So, let's talk about the **importance of strong relationships** and how to **build a support system** that works for you.

Pro Tip: Invest in your relationships. Make time for the people who matter most to you, whether it's family, friends, or even your furry companions. And don't be afraid to reach out and ask for help when you need it—we all need a little support sometimes.

The Friendship Formula: Building Meaningful Connections

Friendships are a **key component** of social health. They provide a sense of belonging, support, and connection that can enhance your overall well-being and resilience. So, let's talk about the **friendship formula** and how to **build meaningful connections** with others.

The Quality over Quantity Principle

When it comes to friendships, **quality is more important than quantity**. It's better to have a few close friends who you can count on than a hundred acquaintances who you barely know. So, let's talk about the **quality over quantity principle** and how to **build meaningful friendships**.

Pro Tip: Focus on quality friendships. Look for people who share your values, interests, and passions. And don't be afraid to be selective—it's better to have a few close friends who you can count on than a hundred acquaintances who you barely know.

The Art of Active Listening: Building Strong Connections

Active listening is a **powerful tool** for building strong and meaningful friendships. It involves paying attention, showing empathy, and providing feedback. So, let's talk about the

art of active listening and how to **build strong connections** with others.

Pro Tip: Practice active listening. Pay attention to what others are saying, show empathy, and provide feedback. And don't forget to **ask questions**—showing genuine interest in others is a great way to build strong and meaningful connections.

The Power of Shared Experiences: Bonding Through Activities

Shared experiences are a **great way** to build strong and meaningful friendships. They provide a sense of connection, belonging, and shared history that can enhance your overall well-being and resilience. So, let's talk about the **power of shared experiences** and how to **bond through activities**.

Pro Tip: Engage in shared experiences with your friends. Whether it's going on a hike, taking a class together, or simply sharing a meal, engaging in activities with others is a great way to build strong and meaningful connections.

The Family Factor: Strengthening Your Closest Bonds

Family is a **crucial component** of social health. It provides a sense of belonging, support, and connection that can enhance your overall well-being and resilience. So, let's talk about the **family factor** and how to **strengthen your closest bonds**.

The Communication Key: Building Strong Family Relationships

Communication is **key** to building strong and meaningful family relationships. It involves listening, expressing yourself clearly, and resolving conflicts in a healthy and constructive way. So, let's talk about the **communication key** and how to **build strong family relationships**.

Pro Tip: Practice open and honest communication with your family. Listen actively, express yourself clearly, and resolve conflicts in a healthy and constructive way. And don't forget to **show appreciation**—letting your family know how much you value them is a great way to strengthen your bonds.

The Quality Time Quotient: Making Memories Together

Quality time is a **crucial component** of strong and meaningful family relationships. It provides a sense of connection, belonging, and shared history that can enhance your overall well-being and resilience. So, let's talk about the **quality time quotient** and how to **make memories together**.

Pro Tip: Spend quality time with your family. Whether it's going on a vacation, having a family game night, or simply sharing a meal together, spending quality time with your family is a great way to build strong and meaningful connections.

The Support System: Being There for Each Other

Support is a **key component** of strong and meaningful family relationships. It involves being there for each other, providing emotional and practical support, and celebrating each other's successes. So, let's talk about the **support system** and how to **be there for each other**.

Pro Tip: Be there for your family. Provide emotional and practical support, celebrate each other's successes, and be a source of comfort and encouragement. And don't forget to **ask for help** when you need it—we all need a little support sometimes.

The Community Connection: Finding Your Tribe

Community is a **powerful force** when it comes to social health. It provides a sense of belonging, support, and connection that can enhance your overall well-being and resilience. So, let's talk about the **community connection** and how to **find your tribe**.

The Power of Belonging: The Importance of Community

Belonging is a **basic human need**. It's the feeling of being seen, heard, and valued by others. And it's a crucial component of overall well-being and resilience. So, let's talk about the **power of belonging** and the **importance of community**.

Pro Tip: Find your tribe. Look for communities that align with your values, interests, and passions. Whether it's a local club, a volunteer group, or an online community, finding your tribe can provide a sense of belonging, support, and connection that enhances your overall well-being and resilience.

The Volunteer Vibe: Giving Back and Connecting

Volunteering is a **great way** to connect with your community and build strong and meaningful relationships. It provides a sense of purpose, belonging, and connection that can enhance your overall well-being and resilience. So, let's talk about the **volunteer vibe** and how to **give back and connect**.

Pro Tip: Volunteer in your community. Look for opportunities that align with your values, interests, and passions. Whether it's helping out at a local food bank, mentoring a child, or cleaning up a park, volunteering is a great way to connect with your community and build strong and meaningful relationships.

The Club and Group Gathering: Finding Your People

Clubs and groups are a **great way** to connect with like-minded individuals and build strong and meaningful relationships. They provide a sense of belonging, support, and connection that can enhance your overall well-being and resilience. So, let's talk about the **club and group gathering** and how to **find your people**.

Pro Tip: Join a club or group that aligns with your values, interests, and passions. Whether it's a book club, a hiking group, or a cooking class, joining a club or group is a great way to connect with like-minded individuals and build strong and meaningful relationships.

The Digital Dinosaur: Navigating Online Connections

The digital world is a **powerful tool** for connecting with others and building strong and meaningful relationships. But it also comes with its own set of challenges and pitfalls. So, let's talk about the **digital dinosaur** and how to **navigate online connections**.

The Social Media Maze: Building Meaningful Connections Online

Social media is a **great way** to connect with others and build strong and meaningful relationships. But it can also be a maze of distractions, comparisons, and superficial interactions. So, let's talk about the **social media maze** and how to **build meaningful connections online**.

Pro Tip: Use social media intentionally. Be mindful of who you connect with, what you share, and how you engage. And don't forget to **set boundaries**—it's okay to take a break from social media and prioritize your offline relationships.

The Online Community Connection: Finding Your Digital Tribe

Online communities are a **great way** to connect with like-minded individuals and build strong and meaningful relationships. They provide a sense of belonging, support, and connection that can enhance your overall well-being and resilience. So, let's talk about the **online community connection** and how to **find your digital tribe**.

Pro Tip: Join online communities that align with your values, interests, and passions. Whether it's a Facebook group, a Reddit forum, or an online course, joining online communities is a great way to connect with like-minded individuals and build strong and meaningful relationships.

The Digital Detox: Balancing Online and Offline Connections

Balancing online and offline connections is **crucial** for overall well-being and resilience. It involves setting boundaries, prioritizing face-to-face interactions, and taking breaks from the digital world. So, let's talk about the **digital detox** and how to **balance online and offline connections**.

Pro Tip: Take a digital detox. Set aside time each day or week to disconnect from the digital world and prioritize your offline relationships. And don't forget to **set boundaries**—it's okay to say no to constant notifications and endless scrolling.

The Romantic Rendezvous: Building Healthy and Fulfilling Relationships

Romantic relationships are a **key component** of social health. They provide a sense of intimacy, connection, and support that can enhance your overall well-being and resilience. So, let's talk about the **romantic rendezvous** and how to **build healthy and fulfilling relationships**.

The Communication Key: Building Strong and Meaningful Connections

Communication is **key** to building strong and meaningful romantic relationships. It involves listening, expressing yourself clearly, and resolving conflicts in a healthy and constructive way. So, let's talk about the **communication key** and how to **build strong and meaningful connections**.

Pro Tip: Practice open and honest communication with your partner. Listen actively, express yourself clearly, and resolve conflicts in a healthy and constructive way. And don't forget to **show appreciation**—letting your partner know how much you value them is a great way to strengthen your connection.

The Quality Time Quotient: Making Memories Together

Quality time is a **crucial component** of strong and meaningful romantic relationships. It provides a sense of connection, belonging, and shared history that can enhance your overall well-being and resilience. So, let's talk about the **quality time quotient** and how to **make memories together**.

Pro Tip: Spend quality time with your partner. Whether it's going on a date, taking a trip together, or simply sharing a meal, spending quality time with your partner is a great way to build strong and meaningful connections.

The Support System: Being There for Each Other

Support is a **key component** of strong and meaningful romantic relationships. It involves being there for each other, providing emotional and practical support, and celebrating each other's successes. So, let's talk about the **support system** and how to **be there for each other**.

Pro Tip: Be there for your partner. Provide emotional and practical support, celebrate each other's successes, and be a source of comfort and encouragement. And don't forget to **ask for help** when you need it—we all need a little support sometimes.

CHAPTER 10: THE FUTURE OF FOSSILS: CUTTING-EDGE SCIENCE FOR DINO LONGEVITY

Alright, folks! We've talked about diet, exercise, stress management, social health, and creating a healthy home environment. Now it's time to dive into the **future of fossils**. Think of this chapter as your ultimate guide to the **cutting-edge science** that's pushing the boundaries of cellular health and longevity. Get ready to geek out on some seriously cool stuff!

The Genomic Revolution: Unlocking the Secrets of Your DNA

The **genomic revolution** is here, and it's changing the game when it comes to understanding and optimizing our health. Let's talk about how **genomic science** is unlocking the secrets of your DNA and paving the way for personalized medicine.

The DNA Deep Dive: Understanding Your Genetic Blueprint

Your DNA is like a **blueprint** for your body. It contains all the instructions needed to make you, well, you. But it's not just a static set of instructions—your DNA is constantly interacting with your environment and lifestyle choices.

Pro Tip: Get to know your DNA. Understanding your genetic blueprint can provide valuable insights into your health risks, strengths, and areas where you can make targeted improvements.

The Epigenetic Enigma: How Your Lifestyle Shapes Your Genes

Epigenetics is the study of how your lifestyle and environment can **turn genes on or off**. It's like the **control panel** for your DNA, determining which genes get expressed and which stay silent.

Pro Tip: Optimize your epigenetics. Lifestyle choices like diet, exercise, stress management, and sleep can all influence your epigenetic profile. By making healthy choices, you can optimize your gene expression and enhance your overall health.

The Personalized Medicine Pioneers: Tailoring Treatments to Your DNA

Personalized medicine is a **game-changer**. It involves tailoring treatments and interventions to your unique genetic makeup. This means more effective, targeted care that's designed just for you.

Pro Tip: Explore personalized medicine. Talk to your doctor about genetic testing and personalized treatment options. Understanding your genetic profile can help guide your healthcare decisions and optimize your outcomes.

The Microbiome Marvel: Harnessing the Power of Your Gut Bacteria

The **microbiome** is the **community of microorganisms** that live in and on your body. These tiny critters play a **huge role** in your overall health, affecting everything from digestion to immune function to even your mood.

The Gut-Brain Connection: How Your Microbiome Influences Your Mind

The **gut-brain axis** is the **two-way communication** between your gut and your brain. It's a complex network of nerves, hormones, and neurotransmitters that allows your gut microbiome to influence your mental health and vice versa.

Pro Tip: Nurture your gut-brain connection. Eat a diet rich in prebiotic and probiotic foods to support a healthy gut microbiome. This can help improve your digestion, boost your immune system, and even enhance your mental health.

The Probiotic Power-Up: Enhancing Your Microbiome with Beneficial Bacteria

Probiotics are **live bacteria** that can **benefit your health**. They help restore the balance of good bacteria in your gut, improve digestion, boost your immune system, and even reduce inflammation.

Pro Tip: Incorporate probiotics into your diet. Foods like yogurt, kefir, sauerkraut, kimchi, and kombucha are great sources of probiotics. You can also consider taking a probiotic supplement to enhance your gut health.

The Prebiotic Push: Feeding Your Good Bacteria

Prebiotics are **non-digestible food ingredients** that **feed the good bacteria** in your gut. They help promote the growth of beneficial microorganisms, enhancing your overall gut health.

Pro Tip: Eat prebiotic foods. Foods rich in prebiotics include fruits, vegetables, whole grains, and legumes. Incorporating these foods into your diet can help support a healthy gut microbiome and enhance your overall health.

The Stem Cell Saga: Regenerative Medicine and the Quest for Longevity

Stem cells are the **building blocks** of your body. They have the **unique ability** to transform into different types of cells, making them a powerful tool for regenerative medicine.

The Regenerative Medicine Revolution: Healing from Within

Regenerative medicine is a **cutting-edge field** that focuses on **healing and regenerating** damaged tissues and organs. It uses stem cells, biomaterials, and other innovative technologies to promote healing and restore function.

Pro Tip: Explore regenerative medicine. Talk to your doctor about regenerative medicine options for conditions like joint pain, tissue damage, and even organ failure. This field is rapidly advancing and offers exciting possibilities for healing and longevity.

The Stem Cell Therapy: Harnessing the Power of Regeneration

Stem cell therapy involves using **stem cells** to **repair and regenerate** damaged tissues. It's a promising approach for treating a wide range of conditions, from arthritis to heart disease to even neurological disorders.

Pro Tip: Consider stem cell therapy. If you're dealing with a condition that could benefit from regenerative medicine, talk to your doctor about stem cell therapy options. This treatment can help promote healing, reduce inflammation, and enhance your overall health.

The Ethical Dilemma: Navigating the Complexities of Stem Cell Research

Stem cell research is a **complex and controversial** field. It raises ethical questions about the use of embryonic stem cells, the potential for cloning, and the regulation of research and therapies.

Pro Tip: Stay informed about stem cell research. Keep up-to-date with the latest developments and ethical debates in the field. Understanding the complexities of stem cell research can help you make informed decisions about your healthcare.

The Nanotechnology Nexus: Tiny Tech with Big Potential

Nanotechnology is the **science of the very small**. It involves manipulating matter at the atomic and molecular level to create new materials and devices with unique properties.

The Nanomedicine Marvel: Revolutionizing Healthcare at the Molecular Level

Nanomedicine is the **application of nanotechnology** to healthcare. It involves using **nanoscale materials** to diagnose, treat, and prevent diseases. This field has the potential to revolutionize healthcare by enabling more precise and effective treatments.

Pro Tip: Explore nanomedicine. Talk to your doctor about nanomedicine options for conditions like cancer, infectious diseases, and even genetic disorders. This field is rapidly advancing and offers exciting possibilities for targeted and personalized healthcare.

The Nanobots: Tiny Robots with Big Potential

Nanobots are **tiny robots** designed to perform specific tasks at the cellular level. They have the potential to revolutionize healthcare by enabling precise and targeted interventions.

Pro Tip: Stay tuned for nanobots. While still in the early stages of development, nanobots hold great promise for the future of healthcare. Keep an eye on this field as it continues to advance and offer new possibilities for diagnosis and treatment.

The Ethical Considerations: Navigating the Complexities of Nanotechnology

Nanotechnology raises **complex ethical questions** about the potential risks and benefits of manipulating matter at the atomic and molecular level. It's important to consider these issues as the field continues to advance.

Pro Tip: Stay informed about nanotechnology. Keep up-to-date with the latest developments and ethical debates in the field. Understanding the complexities of nanotechnology can help you make informed decisions about your healthcare.

The AI Advantage: Harnessing Artificial Intelligence for Health

Artificial intelligence (AI) is **transforming healthcare** by enabling more precise, personalized, and efficient care. Let's talk about how AI is harnessing the power of data to enhance our health and well-being.

The Data-Driven Diagnosis: Using AI to Improve Healthcare Outcomes

AI is revolutionizing healthcare by enabling **data-driven diagnosis**. It uses machine learning algorithms to analyze vast amounts of data and identify patterns and insights that can improve healthcare outcomes.

Pro Tip: Embrace data-driven diagnosis. Talk to your doctor about AI-powered diagnostic tools that can help identify health issues early and guide treatment decisions. This technology has the potential to enhance the accuracy and efficiency of healthcare.

The Personalized Medicine Promise: Tailoring Treatments with AI

AI is enabling **personalized medicine** by analyzing genetic data, lifestyle factors, and health history to tailor treatments to individual needs. This means more effective, targeted care that's designed just for you.

Pro Tip: Explore personalized medicine with AI. Talk to your doctor about AI-powered tools that can help guide your healthcare decisions and optimize your outcomes. Understanding your unique health profile can help you make informed choices about your care.

The Ethical Dilemma: Navigating the Complexities of AI in Healthcare

AI in healthcare raises **complex ethical questions** about data privacy, algorithmic bias, and the potential for misuse. It's important to consider these issues as the field continues to advance.

Pro Tip: Stay informed about AI in healthcare. Keep up-to-date with the latest developments and ethical debates in the field. Understanding the complexities of AI in healthcare can help you make informed decisions about your care.

The Wearable Tech Wave: Monitoring Your Health in Real-Time

Wearable technology is **transforming healthcare** by enabling real-time monitoring of health metrics. Let's talk about how wearable tech is helping us stay informed and proactive about our health.

The Fitness Tracker Frenzy: Monitoring Your Activity and Sleep

Fitness trackers are **popular wearable devices** that monitor
your activity levels, sleep patterns, and other health metrics.
They provide valuable insights into your daily habits and
can help you make informed decisions about your health.

Pro Tip: Invest in a fitness tracker. Use it to monitor your
activity levels, sleep patterns, and other health metrics. This
information can help you make informed decisions about
your lifestyle and optimize your overall health.

The Smartwatch Revolution: Staying Connected and Informed

Smartwatches are **versatile wearable devices** that offer a
range of health-monitoring features, from heart rate
tracking to fall detection to even ECG readings. They
provide valuable insights into your health and can help you
stay connected and informed.

Pro Tip: Consider a smartwatch. Use it to monitor your health
metrics and stay connected to important information.
Smartwatches can help you stay informed about your
health and make proactive decisions about your care.

The Ethical Considerations: Navigating the Complexities of Wearable Tech

Wearable technology raises **complex ethical questions**
about data privacy, accuracy, and the potential for
misuse. It's important to consider these issues as the field
continues to advance.

Pro Tip: Stay informed about wearable tech. Keep up-to-
date with the latest developments and ethical debates in
the field. Understanding the complexities of wearable tech
can help you make informed decisions about your health
and privacy.

CHAPTER 11: YOUR DINO LEGACY: PASSING THE TORCH TO THE NEXT GENERATION

Alright, folks! We've talked about diet, exercise, stress management, social health, creating a healthy home environment, and the cutting-edge science of longevity. Now it's time to dive into the **legacy** you leave behind. Think of this chapter as your ultimate guide to **passing the torch** to the next generation and ensuring that your **dino legacy** lives on.

The Importance of Legacy: Why It Matters

Your legacy is about more than just what you leave behind—it's about the **impact** you have on the world and the people around you. It's about the values, lessons, and wisdom you pass down to future generations. So, let's talk about why **legacy matters** and how to **create a lasting impact**.

The Ripple Effect: How Your Actions Shape the Future

Every action you take has a **ripple effect**. It influences not just your own life but also the lives of those around you. Your choices, behaviors, and values can shape the future in profound ways.

Pro Tip: Be mindful of your actions. Understand that every decision you make has the potential to influence others and shape the future. By being intentional and thoughtful, you can create a positive ripple effect that extends far beyond your own life.

The Power of Example: Leading by Example

One of the most powerful ways to create a lasting legacy is by **leading by example**. Your actions speak louder than words, and by living your values, you can inspire others to do the same.

Pro Tip: Live your values. Whether it's through your work ethic, your commitment to family, or your dedication to community service, leading by example is a powerful way to create a lasting impact.

The Wisdom of Experience: Sharing Your Knowledge

Your experiences and the wisdom you've gained over the years are **invaluable**. Sharing this knowledge with others can help guide them, inspire them, and equip them to navigate their own journeys.

Pro Tip: Share your wisdom. Whether it's through mentoring, writing, or simply having meaningful conversations, sharing your experiences and insights can have a profound impact on others.

The Family Legacy: Building Strong and Lasting Bonds

Family is the **foundation** of your legacy. The values, traditions, and bonds you create within your family can shape generations to come. So, let's talk about how to **build a strong and lasting family legacy**.

The Value of Traditions: Creating Meaningful Family Rituals

Traditions are a **powerful way** to create a sense of belonging, connection, and continuity within your family. They can help pass down values, stories, and memories from one generation to the next.

Pro Tip: Establish family traditions. Whether it's a weekly family dinner, an annual vacation, or a special holiday ritual, creating meaningful traditions can help strengthen family bonds and create lasting memories.

The Art of Storytelling: Passing Down Family History

Storytelling is a **timeless art** that can help pass down family history, values, and wisdom. Sharing stories about your ancestors, your own experiences, and the lessons you've learned can help future generations understand their roots and find their place in the world.

Pro Tip: Tell family stories. Share tales of your ancestors, your own adventures, and the lessons you've learned. Storytelling is a powerful way to pass down family history and values.

The Importance of Quality Time: Building Strong Relationships

Spending quality time with your family is **crucial** for building strong and lasting relationships. It provides a sense of connection, belonging, and shared history that can enhance your overall well-being and resilience.

Pro Tip: Make time for family. Whether it's through shared meals, family outings, or simply spending time together at home, investing in quality time with your family can help build strong and lasting relationships.

The Community Legacy: Making a Difference in Your Neighborhood

Your community is an **extension** of your family. It's the place where you live, work, and play, and it's a crucial part of your legacy. So, let's talk about how to **make a difference** in your neighborhood and create a lasting community legacy.

The Power of Volunteering: Giving Back to Your Community

Volunteering is a **great way** to give back to your community and make a positive impact. It provides a sense of purpose, belonging, and connection that can enhance your overall well-being and resilience.

Pro Tip: Volunteer in your community. Look for opportunities that align with your values, interests, and passions. Whether it's helping out at a local food bank, mentoring a child, or cleaning up a park, volunteering is a great way to give back and make a difference.

The Importance of Advocacy: Standing Up for What You Believe In

Advocacy is about **standing up** for what you believe in and working to create positive change in your community. It involves raising awareness, influencing policy, and supporting causes that matter to you.

Pro Tip: Be an advocate. Stand up for what you believe in and work to create positive change in your community. Whether it's through raising awareness, influencing policy, or supporting causes that matter to you, advocacy is a powerful way to make a difference.

The Value of Mentorship: Guiding the Next Generation

Mentorship is a **powerful tool** for guiding the next generation and helping them reach their full potential. It involves sharing your knowledge, experience, and wisdom to support and inspire others.

Pro Tip: Be a mentor. Share your knowledge, experience, and wisdom with the next generation. Whether it's through formal mentorship programs, informal guidance, or simply being a positive role model, mentorship is a powerful way to guide and inspire others.

The Professional Legacy: Leaving Your Mark in the Workplace

Your professional life is a **significant part** of your legacy. It's where you spend a large portion of your time, and it's a place where you can make a lasting impact. So, let's talk about how to **leave your mark** in the workplace and create a professional legacy that endures.

The Importance of Integrity: Building a Reputation of Honesty and Trust

Integrity is the **foundation** of a strong professional legacy. It involves being honest, trustworthy, and ethical in all your actions and decisions. Building a reputation of integrity can help you earn the respect and trust of your colleagues and clients.

Pro Tip: Act with integrity. Be honest, trustworthy, and ethical in all your actions and decisions. Building a reputation of integrity can help you earn the respect and trust of your colleagues and clients.

The Value of Expertise: Becoming a Thought Leader in Your Field

Expertise is a **key component** of a strong professional legacy. It involves developing deep knowledge and skills in your field and becoming a recognized authority. Sharing your expertise can help guide and inspire others and leave a lasting impact.

Pro Tip: Develop your expertise. Continuously learn and grow in your field. Share your knowledge and insights with others to become a thought leader and leave a lasting impact.

The Power of Collaboration: Building Strong Professional Relationships

Collaboration is a **crucial aspect** of a strong professional legacy. It involves working effectively with others, building strong relationships, and creating a supportive and inclusive work environment.

Pro Tip: Collaborate effectively. Build strong relationships with your colleagues, work effectively as a team, and create a supportive and inclusive work environment. Collaboration is a powerful way to leave a lasting impact in the workplace.

The Financial Legacy: Planning for the Future

Your financial legacy is about more than just money—it's about **planning for the future** and ensuring that your loved ones are taken care of. So, let's talk about how to **create a financial legacy** that provides security and peace of mind.

The Importance of Financial Planning: Preparing for the Unexpected

Financial planning is **crucial** for creating a secure and stable future. It involves setting goals, managing your money, and preparing for the unexpected. A solid financial plan can provide peace of mind and ensure that your loved ones are taken care of.

Pro Tip: Create a financial plan. Set goals, manage your money, and prepare for the unexpected. A solid financial plan can provide peace of mind and ensure that your loved ones are taken care of.

The Value of Insurance: Protecting Your Assets and Loved Ones

Insurance is a **key component** of a strong financial legacy. It provides protection for your assets and loved ones in the event of unexpected events like illness, injury, or death. Having the right insurance coverage can provide peace of mind and financial security.

Pro Tip: Get the right insurance. Review your insurance coverage to ensure that you have the protection you need for your assets and loved ones. Having the right insurance can provide peace of mind and financial security.

The Power of Investing: Growing Your Wealth Over Time

Investing is a **powerful tool** for growing your wealth over time. It involves putting your money to work in assets that have the potential to generate returns. Smart investing can help you build a secure financial future and leave a lasting legacy.

Pro Tip: Invest wisely. Diversify your portfolio, seek professional advice, and stay informed about market trends. Smart investing can help you build a secure financial future and leave a lasting legacy.

The Environmental Legacy: Caring for the Planet

Your environmental legacy is about the **impact** you have on the planet and the actions you take to protect and preserve it for future generations. So, let's talk about how to **create an environmental legacy** that makes a difference.

The Importance of Sustainability: Living in Harmony with Nature

Sustainability is about **living in harmony** with nature and ensuring that our actions do not harm the environment. It involves making conscious choices about how we use resources, reduce waste, and protect ecosystems.

Pro Tip: Live sustainably. Make conscious choices about how you use resources, reduce waste, and protect ecosystems. Living in harmony with nature can help create a sustainable future for all.

The Power of Conservation: Protecting Our Natural Resources

Conservation is about **protecting our natural resources** and ensuring that they are available for future generations. It involves taking actions to preserve habitats, protect wildlife, and conserve water and energy.

Pro Tip: Conserve resources. Take actions to preserve habitats, protect wildlife, and conserve water and energy. Conservation is a powerful way to protect our natural resources and ensure they are available for future generations.

The Value of Education: Raising Awareness and Inspiring Action

Education is a **key component** of creating an environmental legacy. It involves raising awareness about environmental issues, inspiring action, and equipping others with the knowledge and skills to make a difference.

Pro Tip: Educate others. Raise awareness about environmental issues, inspire action, and equip others with the knowledge and skills to make a difference. Education is a powerful way to create an environmental legacy that makes a difference.

AFTERWORD: THE DINO'S JOURNEY CONTINUES

Alright, folks! We've covered a lot of ground in this book. From the basics of cellular preservation to the cutting-edge science of longevity, we've explored the many ways you can keep your inner dinosaur roaring and thriving. But here's the thing—the journey doesn't end here. In fact, it's just beginning.

The Never-Ending Quest for Health and Well-Being

The quest for health and well-being is a **never-ending journey**. It's not something you achieve once and then coast on. It's a continuous process of learning, growing, and adapting. Just like our prehistoric ancestors, we need to stay agile, resilient, and always ready to evolve.

Embracing Change and Growth

One of the most important things to remember is that **change is inevitable**. Whether it's changes in your diet, exercise routine, or even your social circle, life is full of twists and turns. The key is to embrace these changes and use them as opportunities for growth.

Pro Tip: Be open to change. See every new challenge as a chance to learn and grow. Whether it's trying a new workout, exploring a different diet, or making new friends, embracing change can lead to incredible personal growth.

The Power of Continuous Learning

Continuous learning is a **crucial part** of the journey. The world of health and well-being is constantly evolving, with new research, technologies, and insights emerging all the time. Staying informed and up-to-date can help you make better decisions and optimize your health.

Pro Tip: Stay curious. Read books, attend workshops, and follow experts in the field. The more you learn, the better equipped you'll be to navigate the complexities of health and well-being.

The Importance of Community

Building a supportive community is **essential** for your journey. Whether it's friends, family, or like-minded individuals, having a network of people who share your values and goals can provide encouragement, motivation, and a sense of belonging.

Pro Tip: Build your tribe. Surround yourself with people who inspire and support you. Join clubs, groups, or online communities that align with your interests and values. A strong community can be a powerful source of strength and resilience.

The Future of Health and Well-Being

The future of health and well-being is **exciting and full of promise**. With advancements in technology, science, and medicine, we have more tools than ever to optimize our health and extend our lifespan. But it's not just about living longer—it's about living better.

The Role of Technology

Technology is playing an **increasingly important role** in health and well-being. From wearable devices that track our health metrics to AI-powered diagnostic tools, technology is revolutionizing how we approach healthcare.

Pro Tip: Embrace technology. Use wearable devices, health apps, and other tech tools to monitor your health and make informed decisions. Technology can be a powerful ally in your quest for optimal health.

The Promise of Personalized Medicine

Personalized medicine is the **wave of the future**. It involves tailoring treatments and interventions to your unique genetic makeup, lifestyle, and health history. This means more effective, targeted care that's designed just for you.

Pro Tip: Explore personalized medicine. Talk to your doctor about genetic testing and personalized treatment options. Understanding your unique health profile can help you make informed decisions and optimize your outcomes.

The Power of Prevention

Prevention is **key** to a long and healthy life. By taking proactive steps to maintain your health, you can avoid many of the chronic diseases and health issues that plague so many people.

Pro Tip: Focus on prevention. Regular check-ups, healthy lifestyle choices, and early intervention can help you stay ahead of health issues and maintain optimal well-being.

The Legacy You Leave Behind

Your legacy is about more than just what you leave behind—it's about the **impact** you have on the world and the people around you. It's about the values, lessons, and wisdom you pass down to future generations.

The Importance of Mentorship

Mentorship is a **powerful way** to leave a lasting legacy. By sharing your knowledge, experience, and wisdom with others, you can guide and inspire them to reach their full potential.

Pro Tip: Be a mentor. Share your knowledge, experience, and wisdom with the next generation. Whether it's through formal mentorship programs, informal guidance, or simply being a positive role model, mentorship is a powerful way to leave a lasting impact.

The Value of Storytelling

Storytelling is a **timeless art** that can help pass down family history, values, and wisdom. Sharing stories about your ancestors, your own experiences, and the lessons you've learned can help future generations understand their roots and find their place in the world.

Pro Tip: Tell family stories. Share tales of your ancestors, your own adventures, and the lessons you've learned. Storytelling is a powerful way to pass down family history and values.

The Power of Example

One of the most powerful ways to create a lasting legacy is by **leading by example**. Your actions speak louder than words, and by living your values, you can inspire others to do the same.

Pro Tip: Live your values. Whether it's through your work ethic, your commitment to family, or your dedication to community service, leading by example is a powerful way to create a lasting impact.

ABOUT THE AUTHOR: YOUR RESIDENT DINO EXPERT

Alright, folks! You've just finished a wild ride through the world of cellular preservation, dinosaur health, and the quest for longevity. But who's the mastermind behind this epic journey? Let me introduce myself—your resident dino expert!

The Dino Whisperer

First things first, I'm not your average health guru. I'm more like a **dino whisperer**, someone who's deeply fascinated by the ancient wisdom of our prehistoric ancestors and how it can apply to our modern lives. I believe that by tapping into the strength, resilience, and adaptability of dinosaurs, we can unlock our own inner power and live healthier, happier lives.

The Journey Begins

My journey into the world of health and well-being started way back when I was just a kid. I was always curious about how things worked, especially when it came to the human body. I spent hours poring over encyclopedias (remember those?), watching nature documentaries, and even dissecting the occasional frog in biology class.

But it wasn't until I stumbled upon the world of paleontology that I truly found my calling. Dinosaurs, with their incredible strength and adaptability, became my obsession. I started to see parallels between their survival strategies and the challenges we face in our modern world. And that's when the lightbulb went off—what if we could apply the wisdom of dinosaurs to our own health and well-being?

The Dino Diet

One of the first things I explored was the **dino diet**. I started looking at what dinosaurs ate and how their diets might have contributed to their strength and longevity. This led me to experiment with my own diet, focusing on whole foods, plenty of plants, and lean proteins. The results were astonishing—I felt more energetic, my skin glowed, and I even started to see improvements in my overall health.

The Fitness Factor

Next, I turned my attention to **fitness**. Dinosaurs were incredibly agile and strong, so I started incorporating more dynamic and functional movements into my workout routine. I ditched the boring treadmill sessions and started doing things like sprints, agility drills, and strength training. Again, the results were amazing—I felt stronger, more flexible, and ready to take on anything.

The Mind-Body Connection

But it wasn't just about the physical stuff. I also started exploring the **mind-body connection**. Dinosaurs had to be incredibly mindful and aware of their surroundings to survive. So, I started practicing mindfulness and meditation, focusing on being present and reducing stress. This had a profound impact on my mental health and overall well-being.

The Social Dinosaur

Finally, I realized that **social connections** were just as important as physical health. Dinosaurs often lived in groups, relying on each other for support and protection. So, I started focusing on building strong, meaningful relationships with friends, family, and community. This sense of belonging and connection has been crucial in maintaining my overall happiness and resilience.

The Dino Legacy

Throughout my journey, I've come to understand that the wisdom of dinosaurs isn't just about physical health—it's about creating a **legacy** that lasts. It's about the values, lessons, and wisdom we pass down to future generations. That's why I'm so passionate about sharing what I've learned with others.

The Power of Sharing

I believe that **sharing knowledge** is one of the most powerful ways to create a lasting impact. That's why I've written this book—to share the insights and strategies I've discovered on my journey. I hope that by reading these pages, you'll be inspired to embrace your own inner dinosaur and live a life that's vibrant, fulfilling, and full of purpose.

The Future of Fossils

The future of health and well-being is **exciting and full of promise**. With advancements in technology, science, and medicine, we have more tools than ever to optimize our health and extend our lifespan. But it's not just about living longer—it's about living better. It's about embracing the journey, staying curious, and always striving to be the best version of yourself.